The Allergy Handbook

An easy-to-read handy reference book on the complex subject of allergies, with the most up-to-date information on what is available in the allergy treatment field, and including lots of practical advice on how to help yourself.

'A comprehensive self-help guide for the layman'— *Journal of Institute of Health Education*

'A clear, comprehensive and easy-to-read introduction to this exciting field of medicine' — *Irish News*

The Allergy Handbook

A doctor's guide to successful treatment

by
Keith Mumby
M.B., Ch.B.

THORSONS PUBLISHING GROUP

First published September 1988

British Library Cataloguing in Publication Data

Mumby, Keith
  The allergy handbook: a doctor's guide to
  successful treatment..
  1. Man. Allergies. Therapy
  I. Title
  616.97'06

ISBN 0-7225-1657-6

Published by Thorsons Publishers Limited,
Wellingborough, Northamptonshire, NN8 2RQ, England

Printed in Great Britain by Billing & Sons Limited, Worcester

10 9 8 7 6 5 4

Contents

Introduction

Most people, even those not directly involved through personal or family illness, have some awareness of the controversy presently surrounding the subject of allergy, and it becomes very confusing for the ordinary man in the street when the medical profession seems split.

Some doctors are arguing that the allergy phenomenon is rare, relates to few illnesses and concerns substances such as food only very exceptionally. Only a few foods are admitted as the cause of allergies, such as gluten (in wheat), milk, eggs, fish (including shellfish), nuts and certain fruits such as strawberries.

Other doctors, still in a minority, insist that allergies are very common and lie unsuspected behind many hitherto untreatable conditions such as arthritis, eczema, migraine. In fact, they point eagerly to a whole host of health problems they claim can be provoked (and cured) by allergies. Nor do they limit the foods or substances that can cause such reactions. Any food (or drink) can do it, they say, even non-food substances, such as hairspray, petrol fumes, plastics and, in fact, potentially all chemicals in our environment. Of course, some non-food allergens have never been in dispute, such as dust, dust-mite, danders and fur, pollen, feathers and mould. But the whole range of 'environmental allergens' now claimed is both startling and, if true, rather frightening. It could be that we are irreversibly harming our surroundings, to the detriment of many future generations.

The mood of this debate is far from easygoing. Descriptions such as 'unproven', 'racketeering' (a reference to the fact that most advanced allergy clinics so far are private organizations), 'dangerous' and 'quackery', abound on one side; 'reactionary', 'drug-oriented', 'narrow-minded', 'unscientific' and 'incompetent', says the other.

In the face of this controversy, it is small wonder that people are confused and uncertain where to turn for help. It is hoped that this book will give you the reader a much clearer idea of where the truth lies, and you will at least be able to understand the arguments better. More than that, it is an instructional manual intended to assist you in getting the kind of help you might need, and which for the time being at least, the medical profession isn't likely to offer you. Once you have learnt what is truth and what is fiction, nothing can shake that knowledge. Ask anyone who has got rid of disabling chronic illness by avoiding milk or some other common food and *they* will tell you about food allergies.

The media, naturally, enjoy a good ding-dong battle — they couldn't sell newspapers otherwise (at least that's what they appear to think). While deploring the deliberate propagation of argument and controversy, perhaps an open public debate is the only way to shake many members of the medical profession out of their apparent indifference and assumed autocracy on health matters. The public, in this instance, have a right to form their own opinion.

After all, we are talking about a suitable diet and a safer lifestyle, not some abstruse medical topic which requires a deep understanding of anatomy and physiology. The trend towards a better, healthier and more ecologically-sound way of living is a movement that should be welcomed by all enlightened health workers. Only those steeped in self-interest (or blind with real ignorance) would fight against it. I could go further and say that medicine itself is facing a revolution.

I believe that the heyday of drugs has passed its peak and that faith in their unlimited efficacy is now rapidly on the wane. Certainly some drugs will always be needed to save lives, but for treating much chronic illness we don't need them and, in my opinion, they are often counter-productive. Their use can create in the physician's mind the totally false notion that a 'treatment' exists when, in fact, it does not. This prevents the search for a real cure.

It is easy for me to turn to many outstanding successes, using methods outlined in this book, and which are often featured by the media. For example, the epileptic who was allergic to wheat (his driving licence was eventually returned to him); the crippled arthritic woman with an allergy to potato who recovered sufficiently to leave her wheelchair and climb a mountain; the unschoolable youth consigned to an institution who was found to have a wheat allergy and turned out happy and normal; the young child who couldn't go out without a cloth tied round his face, now well and normal: there are thousands of others like them in our files in Manchester.

But the fact that these cases have been written up in the daily papers and featured on television, instead of in the *Lancet*, leads most doctors to ignore the stories totally; they are filed away in some drawer of the mind called 'unproven' and then forgotten.

Most people have heard of the Irish boy who I saved from a stiff jail term for grievous bodily harm because I discovered his violent rages were due to an allergy to (of all things) the common potato. Should he have gone to jail and languished? Would it have made sense for me to explain to him that his trouble was a brain reaction to a certain food but that since it wasn't 'scientifically proven' he must go to prison anyway?

Or take the lady who was going blind due to a reaction to house gas (we don't call this an allergy, as such). She has now recovered her vision. Should she have been left to go blind because the debate about allergy hasn't been settled and many doctors would argue that it is not possible to be allergic to house gas? It seems that some doctors would say 'Yes'!

One of the most common criticisms I get is that what we do isn't scientific. It is true that we don't have the same vast research funds at our disposal that the drug industry commands, but some good scientific papers are now available as a result of research done by pioneering allergists. These blaze a trail that others should be eager to follow instead of carping, as is so often the case, on the inadequacies or deficiencies of the study itself.

In the meantime, the intellectual climate gradually improves, largely due to the pressure of public opinion which is forcing doctors to accept facts which they may find unpalatable. It is no longer enough for the average patient to be given a pat on the head and a bottle of pills when he is ill. Far too many patients are now asking questions such as, 'What is the real nature of my illness?'; 'What exactly does this drug do?'; 'What are its side-effects?'; 'Would it be better to change my diet and lifestyle than to continue taking a drug which causes unpleasant symptoms?'. These are awkward questions which expose the weakness of modern impersonal medicine, and I am glad that people are reacting in this way, challenging old dogmas and seeking the truth for themselves.

I repeat that medicine is on the brink of a revolution and I am glad to be a part of it.

In this book you will find evidence of this new exciting approach. Some of the philosophies are my own. The methods have all been pioneered by great men, heroes in the face of savage medical opposition, such as Albert Rowe, Herbert Rinkel, Theron Randolph and Richard Mackarness, to name but a few.

I hope there is enough here to enlighten you, dispel confusion and set your feet on the road to recovery — one to which you are justifiably entitled.

CHAPTER 1

What is allergy?

At the risk of making things too simple, the controversy surrounding allergies can be narrowed down to one word: the definition of the word ALLERGY itself.

When first coined in 1907 this word meant simply 'some foreign substance which causes an unpleasant reaction in the tissue of the body but which doesn't happen to everyone'. For example, an individual might be made sick by drinking milk: clearly this doesn't happen to the majority of people. It is a specific effect, acquired only by certain sensitive individuals. That's an allergy.

Such an effect is obviously different from poisoning. For example, someone who swallowed lysol would probably feel very sick indeed, perhaps even die. But that would happen to everyone. In other words, this effect isn't peculiar or abnormal but a universal cause of tissue damage.

We can start with a basic definition of allergy, then, by saying it is an *unpleasant reaction to foreign matter, specific to that substance, which is altered from the normal response and peculiar to the individual concerned.*

Over the following two decades, researchers showed that the mechanism often involved was a malfunction of the body's immune system. Soon the word 'allergy' came to mean only this sort of response and other reactions, if any, were simply ignored. Not very scientific, you'd probably think, and you would be right.

Disordered immune response

The body has a series of wonderful defence mechanisms, designed to keep us healthy, and without which we would be dead in a matter of hours. One of these we call the immune system. Briefly, it works like this: if a foreign substance such as a bacteria or virus enters the body, the tissues learn to identify the special proteins of the invader and make a chemical antidote which attacks only that specific protein. The attacking (or defending) chemical, manufactured by ourselves, we call an ANTIBODY. The foreign protein it is designed to immobilize, we call the ANTIGEN (Greek suffix -gen: meaning something which creates or causes something to occur).

It is a clever and spectacularly successful system, the detailed complexity of which surpasses our full understanding so far. The main drawback is that the body has to meet the foreign protein (antigen) before it can mobilize its counter-attack (the antibody). In other words, we must be invaded before we can fight back. This may not matter much with an illness like German measles or chicken-pox, but it is a serious inadequacy when it comes to potentially fatal diseases such as smallpox and diphtheria. Basically,

BOX 1

Diagrammatic antigens and antibodies

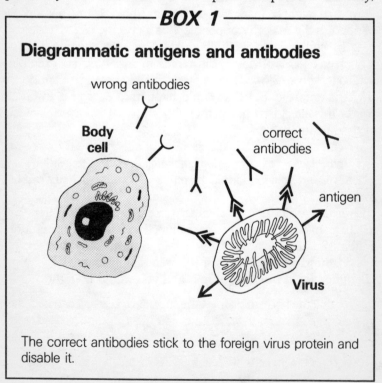

The correct antibodies stick to the foreign virus protein and disable it.

those who survive such dangerous infections do so because their immune systems work very fast and start to produce antibodies in the nick of time, just before death supervenes. Those with a slower immune response are not so lucky and will die.

Or at least they used to. Now we can use vaccination to prevent such deaths. We introduce an artificial infection, commonly done by injecting a dead or weakened virus which does not harm the patient, but teaches his or her body to recognize the virus protein and make antibodies. Thus when the real invaders come along the body is ready and can start its counter-offensive by mobilizing antibodies within hours, instead of days, and so beat off the attack (see Box 1).

White blood cells, particularly lymphocytes, make antibodies. The frightening new disease AIDS (Acquired Immune Deficiency Syndrome) destroys lymphocytes so that the body cannot make antibodies. The victim, therefore, dies of simple everyday infections which can no longer be resisted in the way in which a healthy individual routinely shrugs them off. Ironically, of course, it means also that the body is hampered in its ability to round on the AIDS virus and so this is a particularly grim infection. The search for a vaccine seems very bleak.

Allergy and immunity: the great paradox

I have discussed this topic in some detail because, without understanding immunity, it is hard to understand certain types of allergy reaction. What might be called the conventional view of allergy is based on this mechanism.

It seems that dusts, pollens, foods and other basically harmless substances can act as antigens in some individuals. They enter the body through the lungs or digestive tract and gain access to the tissues where they cause antibodies to be formed. The resulting interaction between antigen and antibody harms the tissues involved and this gives rise to symptoms.

Note that the body must meet the substance before it can become allergic to it: that is, the allergy reaction (symptoms) could only occur on the second or subsequent exposures. Also the symptoms are referred to the organ affected. Pollens and dust affect the eyes (redness and itching) and the nose (catarrh and sneezing). A food allergy will cause abdominal pain, upset and perhaps vomiting or diarrhoea.

The trouble with this glib and satisfying explanation, which conventional allergists defend with a fervour bordering on hysteria, is that it is totally unsupportable. To begin with it doesn't fit the facts. Allergy can have a much more widespread effect than local tissue irritation, as you will see shortly. But more importantly, if you think again about the mechanism described above, you will see that, if it's true, we all should get food or other allergies. In fact we should be continuously sick, if not dead, due to permanent incapacitating reactions to everything we eat and breathe, since all such substances are foreign protein.

Clearly, this is not so and therefore something is wrong with the classic 'explanation' of allergy. Thus the doctors who are clinging most closely to their 'scientific' theories are being the least scientific of all! What they say sounds good, but it is incorrect and is blinding them to the facts.

It was Professor John Soothil who first pointed out this paradox. He is a clever and adventurous thinker, free of many of the strictures that bedevil his conventional colleagues (though, unfortunately, he hasn't much time for doctors like myself who are rebellious and accord no respect to the medical hierarchy!). He was, incidentally, the head of the first team to show incontrovertibly that people can be allergic to foods *without any of the classic criteria or tests for allergy being fulfilled*, thus confirming what a group of doctors around the world have been saying for decades.

Working definition

Having introduced you to the elements of this heated debate, let us now invent our own 'working definition' for the word ALLERGY, and state simply: if you can show that a substance is making someone ill, that reaction is an allergy. Really, that's all that matters so far as the sick individual is concerned. Being healthier means avoiding such substances, so it is essentially a practical definition. It also fits very well with the popular use of the word. The average man or woman in the street doesn't know much about immune disorders, but the concept of 'something to avoid' is simple enough for anyone to grasp.

Of course there must be some way of supporting the assertion that the substance is bad for a person. He or she must be shown to feel better by avoiding it and suffer symptoms when re-exposed to it. To be really sure, the re-exposure test would be done without the patient knowing what to expect. The medical term for this is 'blind' and prevents the patient from colouring the results with opinion or psychological 'reactions'. If the practitioner doesn't know what is being given either — perhaps the substances are coded and the key kept by a third person — we call this 'double-blind'.

Blind challenge tests are all very well for scientific study but not for day-to-day work in a clinic, as it is an unnecessary imposition on the routine. We do not assume the patient will bluff, dissemble, or is feeble minded. This trust seems eminently successful in practice, I'm glad to say!

Once again, I will point out that allergy is not poisoning. Yet the reader will quickly see that a toxic chemical in the environment will fulfil the criteria for the working definition above. Instead of being contradictory, this underlines the value of using a practical concept for the term allergy. In the end, it doesn't matter if the substance is a poison or an allergy: the patient still feels better for avoiding it.

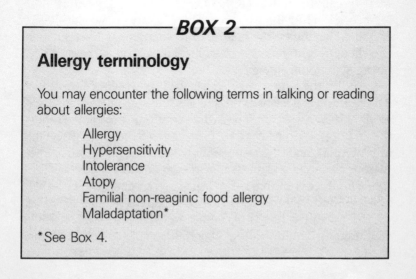

BOX 2

Allergy terminology

You may encounter the following terms in talking or reading about allergies:

> Allergy
> Hypersensitivity
> Intolerance
> Atopy
> Familial non-reaginic food allergy
> Maladaptation*

*See Box 4.

Alternative terms

Other names you may encounter for the allergy phenomenon need not distract us long. IDIOSYNCRACY and HYPERSENSITIVITY are two suggestions. INTOLERANCE has fewer indigestible syllables. Dr Arthur Coca, a famous American allergist spanning the conventional and unconventional, suggested FAMILIAL NON-REAGINIC FOOD ALLERGY. This is somewhat lengthy but conveys the notion that: (a) it tends to run in families (which is true), and (b) antibodies may not be demonstrated. It never caught on, probably because he was decades ahead of his time.

I prefer the term MALADAPTATION SYNDROME, which is explained below (see 'Three stages of allergy'). (See also Box 2.)

But there is no doubt that the most widely known, used and understood label is the one with which we started: ALLERGY.

Now the problem

In actual fact matters are not always so straightforward. It may be possible for someone to be exposed to an allergen (allergic substance) and not experience symptoms if the quantity is below what we call the THRESHOLD DOSE. Only if this critical dose is exceeded will anything happen. This can vary from the tiny traces of pollen floating on the breeze, which makes hay-fever sufferers wretched, to eating several platefuls of a food on successive days before symptoms emerge. (See Box 3.)

Secondly, the patient may not get well by avoiding a substance if there are several allergies present. If someone is allergic to several foods and gives up eating one while continuing to eat the others, this may bring no relief at all. Sometimes there is no detectable improvement until the last offending substance is located, when there is dramatic and sudden cessation of the illness.

Finally, there is one other problem to add confusion — the hidden allergy — and I am convinced it is the main reason that the extent of allergic illness has gone undiscovered for so long. It is the *vital* missing datum, without which the whole subject remains a mystery.

The hidden allergy

An entirely new concept is that of the hidden allergy, first described by Dr Herbert Rinkel. As its name suggests, it makes you ill but you don't know it is doing so. Hidden allergies are far from rare — in fact, they are very common, once you know what to look for. Masked allergy is another expression for the same thing. The masking is almost complete so that the sufferer would never guess correctly from where the trouble is coming. This, of course, makes things terribly difficult.

Anyone can recognize a food allergy when the reaction is acute and the patient flares up in a violent rash each time he or she eats the offending substance. The unlucky sufferer simply avoids the food in question, thus giving rise to the impression that food allergy is rare.

But supposing the allergy is something being eaten every day, or several times a week. The body becomes accustomed to the food in a sickly sort of way, the reaction damps down. Indeed, for many years or even decades, it may seem to disappear altogether, perhaps emerging only occasionally when a little too much is taken at one sitting or some other complicating factor, such as stress, temporarily lowers resistance. Because of the very infrequency of the effect, it is most unlikely that the sufferer will ever recognize the cause of the symptoms.

Eventually, however, resistance runs out. The body can no longer cope and sickness emerges. The final form of the disease suffered may vary greatly from person to person and really depends on what part of the body receives the brunt of the attack (see the section on Target or Shock Organs, in the next chapter).

Not all hidden allergies are foods, but the fact that we become tolerant to such an effect is easy to explain in terms of food. If you eat something to which you are allergic every few days — and as you will see, allergy foods are often consumed daily — it means the body is never really free of this offending substance. As fast as you evacuate it from the bowel, more is introduced into the stomach. Precisely because the body is never completely free of the substance, the new dose doesn't make any significant difference, so it tends not to react. It is very important to understand this point.

In a later chapter, you will be told to avoid a food strictly for a minimum of four days before trying a challenge test by eating it.

This is so that it will clear the bowel and no longer be masked.

Chemicals and other substances can become masked in exactly the same way by frequent exposure. The maximum length of time between doses needed to keep up the masking depends on how rapidly each substance is excreted from the body or detoxified by the liver.

Threshold doses

Another key phenomenon that makes allergy confusing is the concept of threshold doses. It takes a certain quantity of an allergen to trigger a symptom. Below this level, the individual can tolerate the substance and remain quite well. If the allergen is a food, it could mean that person can eat reasonable quantities of the food. Only when indulging it to excess do symptoms appear. Naturally, this can make it very confusing when trying to track down such an allergen. At other times, even the most infinitesimal dose of the allergen sets off a reaction. In other words, the threshold is then very low. Just to make things complicated, thresholds vary from substance to substance in the same individual.

Allergens can also combine in their effect. This could result in symptoms due to a mysterious combination of substances, even though each separate item is incapable of having an effect on its own. This explains the sometimes peculiar behaviour of allergies which so bedevils investigation, if you don't understand what the problem is.

The diagrams in Box 3 should clarify the threshold effect.

Three stages of allergy

Already, then, we can pinpoint three different stages in the allergy process. Stage 1 occurs when the allergy reacts directly on the body. Symptoms are produced. In fact if you have understood everything so far, there has to be a prior step. On first meeting the food nothing unpleasant happens at all, except that the body is sensitized to it and only subsequent to this can an allergy come into being. We can call this Stage 0.

Stage 2 occurs when the body has become accustomed to the allergen. By frequent exposure the reaction is muted. Ill effects

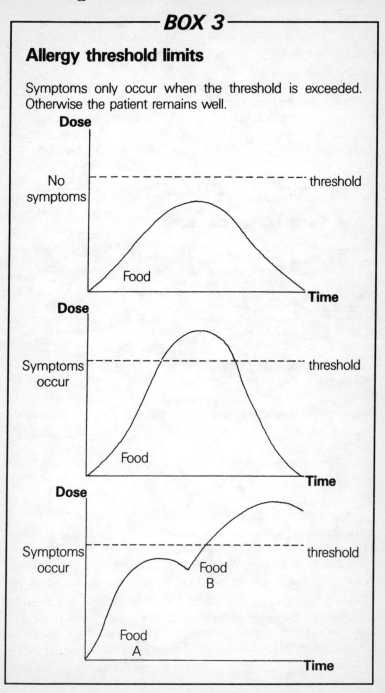

BOX 3

Allergy threshold limits

Symptoms only occur when the threshold is exceeded. Otherwise the patient remains well.

become disguised or masked. For a time there may be no symptoms at all, simply the storing up of trouble. We could call Stage 2 one of *adaptation* to an unhealthy substance.

What happens if the person goes on eating the food? If an individual continues to expose himself to an adapted allergen, eventually the body's ability to resist runs out. At first this may only happen from time to time, say when the person is under stress, but eventually symptoms start up in earnest. We are now in Stage 3 and logically, this is called MALADAPTATION. (See Box 4.)

BOX 4

The three stages of allergy

Stage 1 Alarm stage
Meeting the offending substance causes a symptom.

Stage 2 Adaptation
Frequent exposure to the offending substance accustoms the body to it. Symptoms usually subside.

Stage 3 Maladaptation
The body can no longer cope. Resistance has run out. Symptoms return. This may entail **Addiction,** when symptoms appear to be relieved by intake of the offending substance.

Addiction

Finally, we reach a stage of addiction: the patient craves the food and wants to eat it often, even to binge the food. The reason is that by this stage, ironically, the patient gets the symptoms *only if he or she doesn't eat the food*. We call these withdrawal symptoms. Even a small helping of the allergen in question actually relieves these symptoms.

However, it only appears to improve matters, because eating the food *masks* the symptoms (this is the real meaning of a masked allergy). The truth is that the body is already on the slippery slope to ruin.

Incidentally, one of the reasons alcohol is consumed so liberally in our society is that it readily masks food withdrawal symptoms. Feeling rough? A good stiff drink will soon fix that!

The curious thing is that if you give someone who is craving a drink a dose of pure alcohol, it does no good at all. If, however, you give him or her just a tiny dose of wheat, sugar, yeast, corn or whatever *foodstuff* the person is addicted to, the craving for the drink goes away!

So that's allergy in a nutshell. Now, let us take a look at the effects allergies produce.

CHAPTER 2

The results of allergy

Probably nothing has caused more confusion in respect of recent developments in allergy than the recognition of the multiplicity of symptoms it can produce. No doubt this has hampered progress, since the traditional medical view of patients with many and variable symptoms has always been that they are somehow neurotic and 'putting it all on'.

This dismissive tendency is made worse if the patient has psychological disturbances, yet few doctors have ever thought to question whether such personality changes could *also* be caused by an allergy. Even if it were not so, if you had a chronic disease or symptoms which came and went in a baffling way — headache one week, sore throat the next, diarrhoea the next, and so on — wouldn't you expect to feel bad mentally? It is gross folly, if not arrogance, to say that the *cause* of their illness is their inability to cope well mentally. This is not to say that there are no neurotic individuals whose symptoms are an attempt to win sympathy from a world they find too hostile; merely that such people are in a small minority.

How do such changeable and mysterious symptoms come about? The modern allergist thinks in terms of target organs.

Target organs

Probably the most common question I am asked during radio interviews is which allergies cause which symptoms. Apart from the fact that dust and pollens tend to cause rhinitis, there is no reliable connection. The symptom depends on which part of the body is being attacked, not on what is doing it. Thus, milk allergy, if it affects the nose, will also cause rhinitis. This astonishes patients at first.

The concept is really very simple — we call it the target or shock organ principle. An allergic reaction is, of course, a manifestation of the whole person, but some part of the body, or a particular organ (for reasons which are not clear) receives more of the trauma

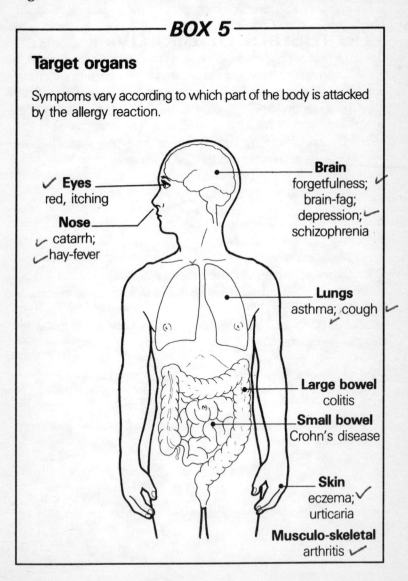

BOX 5

Target organs

Symptoms vary according to which part of the body is attacked by the allergy reaction.

✓ **Eyes**
red, itching

Nose
catarrh;
hay-fever

Brain
forgetfulness;
brain-fag;
depression;
schizophrenia

Lungs
asthma; cough

Large bowel
colitis

Small bowel
Crohn's disease

Skin
eczema;
urticaria

Musculo-skeletal
arthritis

than the rest. Symptoms will depend largely on the function of this organ, which will either be excited (stirred up) or depressed (slowed down).

Thus, an allergy attacking the lungs will cause asthma; one which attacks the bowel will produce abdominal pain, bloating and maybe diarrhoea or vomiting; one which attacks the joints will produce aching and stiffness; one which attacks the head will produce headaches and so on. (See Box 5.)

Undoubtedly, the most sensitive organ in the body is the brain. It is the seat of our highest functions, and thought is easily disturbed. This disturbance can be as mild as forgetfulness, or as frightening as full-blown dementia. Probably the most common symptom of all is what Theron Randolph dubbed the 'woolly brain syndrome' (brain fag), which describes it perfectly. The brain won't think straight — it seems 'foggy' somehow — and it is hard for the patient to concentrate and remember things. This can happen to anyone, even very intelligent people, many of whom rely on their intellect to make a living, such as executives and bankers.

Five key symptoms

You can imagine that the range of potential symptoms caused by allergy is vast. Nevertheless, Dr Richard Mackarness gives five key symptoms which point the way to allergic illness and which have special importance. He believes that without one of the following symptoms diagnosis is unlikely:

- Over- or under-weight or fluctuating weight
- Persistent fatigue that isn't helped by rest
- Occasional swellings around the eyes, hands, abdomen, ankles, etc.
- Palpitations or speeded heart rate, particularly when occurring after meals
- Excessive sweating, not related to exercise

It needs adding that there should be no other explanation for these symptoms. Do any of them apply to you?

A useful table of symptoms

BOX 6

Symptoms commonly associated with maladaptation syndrome

Abdominal bloating
Abrupt change of state
   from well to unwell
Aching muscles
Asthma
Blotches on the skin
Bronchitis
Catarrh
Chest pain
Chilblains
Constipation
Convulsions
Crabby on waking
Cramps in limbs
Diarrhoea
Difficulty waking up
'Dopey' feeling
Dyspepsia, abdominal
   distress
Eating binges
Eczema
Feeling faint
Feeling totally drained and
   exhausted
Feeling unreal,
   depersonalized
Feeling unwell all over
Flatulence
'Flu-like state' that isn't
   'flu
Frequent urination
General slowing down
General speeding up

Giddiness
Headache (including
   migraine)
High blood pressure
High mood (undue
   elation)
Inability to think clearly
Insomnia
Irritability
Itching
Lack of confidence
Low mood
Menstrual difficulties
Mood swings
Mouth ulcers
Nausea
Panic attacks
Rash that is not eczema
Red or itchy eyes
Ringing in the ears
   (tinnitus)
Shaking in the morning
Slow getting started in the
   morning
Stiffness in throat or
   tongue
Stomach pain
Sudden chills and tingling
   after eating
Sudden sneezing
Sudden tiredness after
   eating
Swollen painful joints

BOX 6 (cont)

Terrible thoughts on
  waking
Tingling all over
Unusually slow or rapid
  heartbeat

Variability of bowel
  function
Vomiting without nausea
Water retention

The table in Box 6 lists symptoms commonly associated with maladaptation syndrome. (Note, the list is far from complete.)

The trouble with all such tables is that they may be misleading. Most of the symptoms could be caused by some other illness, although several, admittedly, are peculiar to allergies. What really matters is a spread of symptoms — the more of these you have the more likely it is that your illness is allergic in origin.

Some are quite obvious: those denoting digestive disturbance would point particularly to a food allergy in the absence of any other pathology. Those affecting the brain show up clearly as mood changes, altered feelings, etc. Abrupt changes from well to unwell (well one minute, sick a few hours later) are pretty characteristic of allergic reactions.

What often surprises people are those symptoms of feeling bad first thing in the morning. That is not an allergy, they say, it's so common — it's almost normal to feel that way.

You need to think back to what I said about addiction. By the time a person wakes up in the morning, he or she has often been off food for twelve to fourteen hours: that's enough to start up *withdrawal* symptoms. He or she has breakfast, which acts like a 'fix' of a drug and within an hour or two symptoms disappear! Certainly these feelings are common, but that's only because masked food allergies are very common.

Another surprise is the 'four-day 'flu', which isn't really 'flu at all — it's a food allergy! The person eats the food, the symptoms are centred on the nose and muscles so he or she experiences headache, runny nose, aches and pains, maybe even a temperature, but a few days later, when the food leaves the bowel, the symptoms disappear. That's too quick for the natural course of a virus disease. As Dr Arthur Coca says in *The Pulse Test* (Lyle Stuart, 1982), 'You don't catch colds, you eat them!'

If you have a number of symptoms from the table, but otherwise feel well, you should still consider changing your diet. In doing so you may prevent yourself getting a more serious illness in years to come.

The diseases

Just as we can have a table of symptoms caused by allergy, so we can make a table of diseases (see Box 7). Possibly it will need to be added to as we learn more. I am talking now about the purely empirical approach — in a number of these diseases, for example rheumatoid arthritis, we have no idea what the root cause is, but we are certain from direct practical experience that allergies play a part and the disease can be put into remission, sometimes even cured completely, by a change of diet and environment.

BOX 7

Diseases with a possible allergic basis

Alcoholism
Arthritis (rheumatoid and
    osteo-)
Asthma ✓
Coeliac disease
Colitis
Crohn's disease
Eczema ✓
Haemorrhoids
Hyperkinetic syndrome
Meniere's disease

Migraine ✓
Obesity
Peptic ulcer
Perennial rhinitis (all year ✓
    round)
Polyarteritis nodosa
Polymyaligia rheumatica
Seasonal rhinitis
    (hay-fever)
Temporal arteritis
Urticaria (hives)

Less commonly, the following diseases may have an allergic basis:

Anxiety
Behavioural disorders
Depression
Diabetes
Epilepsy

Mindless (unprovoked)
    violence
Mouth ulcers ✓
Psoriasis
Schizophrenia

At first sight, it seems incredible that so many different conditions can be caused by allergies, but a clearer understanding of the functions of the target organs helps to explain this.

The best discoveries in science, as always, are very simple in scope, wide in application and explain many previous mysteries. Maladaptation to common environmental substances attacking random organs in the body fits this description exactly.

The common allergens

Many doctors, when confronted with an allergy, seem to melt like snowflakes in a blast furnace. 'It could be any one of ten thousand things!' they say, and promptly give up, preferring instead to prescribe a palliative drug (one aimed only at the symptoms, not at the cause) which doesn't tax their powers of observation and deduction.

Fortunately, the truth is very much easier to confront. Almost all reactions come principally from about two dozen substances, of which the majority are foods but also include well-known allergens such as dust, dust-mite and moulds (antibiotics are derived from moulds and these give rise to probably the most common drug reactions).

Several doctors and study centres have worked out league tables of the most frequent offenders and the results are remarkably

---

BOX 8

Most frequent food allergens

Without worrying about the exact order, the table would look as follows:

Beef	Orange
Cane sugar	Pork
Chocolate	Potato
Coffee	Tea
Corn	Tomato
Egg	Wheat
✓ Milk	Yeast

consistent. For adults, wheat always comes out top, followed by milk, with instant coffee, yeast, cheese, sugar, citrus fruit, egg and several others not far behind. (See Box 8.)

For children, the top offenders are corn and chemical additives (wheat is not nearly so common a problem in children). Conversely, chemical food additives are less common offenders in adults, perhaps because our larger and more mature livers can detoxify them relatively easily.

Forearmed with this knowledge it is much easier to track down the source of trouble. It also makes the construction of elimination diets quite simple.

Allergies are not fixed

Some allergy reactions remain unaltered throughout life. Typically, these are the antigen–antibody mediated 'classic' allergies such as shellfish and strawberries (food) or dust and pollens (inhalants), but not always so. The majority of allergies can vary considerably in their effect over a period of time. If you avoid the substance, the reaction tends to die down. If you eat it a lot, the allergy becomes worse.

Thus, you will see that eating the same foods repeatedly tends to provoke trouble and if you look at the table of frequent food allergens shown in Box 8 you will see that they are common foods that some of us eat daily.

So far then, the facts fit the theory. Let us see how we can use this knowledge to bring about a recovery for you and your family.

CHAPTER 3

Elimination dieting

Elimination and challenge dieting may not result in you getting well. This doesn't mean that you don't have allergies, but it may mean that you have simultaneous non-food or, as we term them, environmental allergies.

Even that may not be the whole story. You may have concomitant vitamin and mineral deficiencies, hormone disorders and disturbed bowel bacteria, but more of that in later chapters.

However, we always start our approach with food allergies, not because we are saying that everything is food allergy, but because: (a) it is the easiest to deal with, and (b) often all you need to do is to get rid of offending foods. The body is then able to cope with the remaining allergens, if there are any. (See Box 9.)

BOX 9

Symptoms suggesting food sensitivity

✓Bloating and flatulence
✓Falling asleep after meals
✓Food binges
✓Food cravings
✓Irritable, lethargic or shaky on waking (i.e. before breakfast)
Palpitations related to food
Symptoms after eating
Symptoms relieved by food
✓Weight gain or fluctuations in weight

The secret of successful identification of food allergies is to give up sufficient foods to feel well, then to re-introduce these foods one at a time, so that detecting a reaction is relatively easy. It rarely works to give up just one food at a time because anyone who is ill is almost certain to have more than one allergy. If it was simply one major allergen, the person would have spotted it eventually, as indeed some lucky people do.

The rest of this chapter is given over to discussing three-tiered dieting, from which you can choose the most appropriate approach for you or your family. Let us start with the easiest.

An easy elimination diet (14–21 days)

It is logical to start by eliminating only the common food allergies. This leaves plenty of foods to eat and you should not find this diet too onerous. It is especially suitable for a child and consists basically of fresh meat, fish, fruit and vegetables, with water to drink. We call it the 'Stone-Age diet'. (See Box 10.)

It is vital to understand that you must not cheat on this or any other exclusion diet: to do so could prevent your recovery. Remember that it takes several days for food to clear your bowel. If you do slip up, you will need to extend the avoidance period for several more days. Later on, when the detective work is complete, the occasional indiscretion won't matter. In the meantime, follow the instructions exactly.

Don't forget about addictions. It is quite likely that you will get withdrawal symptoms during the first few days. This is good news because it means you have given up something important. Usually the effects are mild and amount to nothing more than feeling irritable, tired, or perhaps having a headache, but be warned — it could put you in bed for a couple of days.

Please note that it is possible to be allergic even to the allowed foods — they are chosen simply because reaction to them is less common. If you are in this minority, you might even feel worse on this diet, but at least it proves you have a food allergy. In that case, try eliminating, also, the foods you are eating more of (potato is a common offender) and see if you then begin to improve. If not, you should switch to the Eight Foods Diet, or a fast as described below.

DO NOT, simply because you do not improve, make the erroneous assumption that you could not then be allergic to milk,

BOX 10

An easy elimination diet (the 'Stone-Age diet')

NOT ALLOWED	ALLOWED
Milk, butter, cheese, cream, margarine, yogurt, skimmed and goat's milk	Beef, pork and lamb
	Turkey, duck and other fowl
Wheat (including bread, cakes, pasta, etc.), corn, rice, rye, oats, barley, millet	All fish (not smoked)
	Fresh vegetables
Egg, chicken	Fresh fruit (except citrus)
Citrus fruit (orange, lemon, etc.)	Bottled spring water, filtered water
Sugar, honey or sweeteners	Fruit juices
Tea or coffee	Herb teas (avoid 'blends')
Alcoholic drinks	Salt, pepper and herbs
Processed meats or smoked fish	
Any tinned, bottled or packet food	
Tap water	
Tobacco	
Spices, pills, potions and remedies	

Do not stop medical drugs without consulting your doctor.

wheat or other banned foods. This would be a serious mistake which could bar your road to recovery.

By the way, don't worry about special recipes or substitutes at this stage. By the time you have fried, baked, steamed and grilled everything once, the two weeks will almost have passed! If in the long term it transpires that you need to keep off a food, then you can begin searching for an alternative. While on the elimination diet, try to avoid hanging on to a few favourite foods and eating only those. You must eat with variety, otherwise you will risk creating reactions to the foods you are eating repeatedly. It is senseless to go on with old habits. The whole point of exclusion dieting is to make you change what you are doing — it could be making you ill.

A word about drugs

Drug allergies are not rare and it may be wise to discontinue medications which are not necessary. However, certain drugs are essential and should not be stopped, such as antiepileptics, some cardiac drugs (such as digoxin), insulin, thyroxin and others. Some medications, such as cortisone derivatives, need to be phased out gradually.

To be certain, it is better to discuss the implications with your doctor and ask his or her advice on stopping your treatment. Don't be put off by the arrogance which some doctors, sadly, are prone to when their prescriptions are questioned. *You are entitled to know* the effect of any drug you are taking and also precisely *why* you are taking it, and it may be that your doctor will not understand the workings and side-effects of drugs being used.

The key question that you want answered is, 'Will I come to harm if I stop this drug?' Nine times out of ten the answer is, 'No'.

Don't forget, tobacco is a drug. You must stop smoking if you are serious about getting well.

The eight foods diet (7–14 days)

Not as severe as a fast but tougher than the previous regime, is what Professor John Soothil calls the Few Foods Diet. Obviously it is more likely to succeed since you are giving up more foods. Any determined adult could cope with it, but on no account should you subject a child to this diet without his, or her, full and voluntary co-operation. It could produce a severe emotional trauma otherwise. (Factually, there is rarely a problem. Most children don't want to be ill and will assist you, providing they understand what you are trying to do.)

The basic idea is to produce one or two relatively safe foods for each different category we eat. Everyday foods are avoided since these include the common allergens. Thus we would choose fruits such as mango and kiwi, not apple and banana; flesh such as duck and rabbit, not beef and pork. The diet (in Box 11) contains my suggestions. You can vary it somewhat according to what is available to you locally.

━━━ BOX 11 ━━━

The eight foods diet

Allowed foods:

MEAT	Turkey, rabbit
VEGETABLES	Spinach, turnip
FRUIT	Mango, kiwi
CARBOHYDRATES	Buckwheat, millet

Sea salt only for seasoning.

Drink only bottled spring water.

The main problem is boredom. However, there is enough variety here for adequate nourishment over the suggested period, providing you eat a balance of all eight foods. Exotic fruits can be expensive, but you won't need to eat them for long, and, in any case, few people would deny that feeling well is worth any expense.

The chances are that, on a diet like this, you will feel well within a week, but for some conditions, such as eczema and arthritis, you will need to allow a little longer. Be prepared to go the full two weeks before deciding that it isn't working.

The fast (4–7 days)

Although a fast is the ultimate approach in tracking down hidden food allergies, I don't recommend it lightly. It is the fastest way to feeling well, if your illness is caused by food allergy. Thus, although it can be tough at first, by the morning of the fifth day, you will feel wonderful! The real problem is that sometimes it can then be difficult to get back on to any safe foods. Everything is unmasked at once and the patient seems to react to everything he or she tries to eat. This can cause great distress.

Undertake a fast only if you are very determined or you suspect food allergy and the other two approaches have failed.

Fasting is emphatically not suitable for certain categories of patient:

- Pregnant women

- Children

- Diabetics

- Anyone seriously weakened or debilitated by chronic illness

- Anyone who has been subject to severe emotional disturbance (especially those prone to violent outbursts, or those who have tried to commit suicide)

- Epileptics

The fast itself is simple enough — just don't eat for four or five days. Drink only bottled spring water. You must stop smoking. The whole point is to empty your bowels entirely of foodstuffs. Thus, if you have any tendency to constipation, take Epsom salts to begin with. If in doubt try an enema! Otherwise the effort may be wasted.

A variation, which I call the 'half fast', is to eat only two foods, such as lamb and pears. This means taking a gamble that neither lamb nor pears are allergenic, and it is not as sure-fire as the fast proper. It is permissible to carry this out for seven days, but on no account go on for longer than this.

Food challenge testing

As soon as you feel well, you can begin testing, although you must not do so before the four-day unmasking period has elapsed. Allow longer if you have been constipated.

Of course, you may never improve on an elimination diet. The problem may be something else. In that case, when three weeks (maximum) have elapsed on the simple elimination diet, two weeks on the Eight Foods Diet, or seven days on a fast, then you must begin re-introducing foods. This is vital. It is not enough to feel well on a very restricted diet: we want to know why. What are the culprits? These are the foods you must avoid long-term, not all those which are banned at the beginning.

Even if you don't feel well, as already pointed out, this does not prove you have no allergies amongst the foods you gave up. Test the foods as you re-introduce them, anyway — you may be in for a surprise.

The procedure is as follows, except for those coming off a fast:

- Eat a substantial helping of the food, preferably on its own for the first exposure.

- Wait several hours to see if there is an immediate reation, and if not, eat some more of the food, along with an ordinary meal, such as you have been eating.

- You may eat a third, or fourth, portion if you want, to be sure.

- Take your resting pulse (sit still for two minutes) before, and several times during the first 90 minutes after the first exposure to the food. A rise of ten or more beats in the RESTING pulse is a fairly reliable sign of an allergy. If there is no change in the pulse it does not mean the food is safe, unless symptoms are absent also.

- Choose only whole, single foods, not mixtures and recipes. Try to get supplies that have not been chemically treated in any way.

- If you get an unpleasant reaction, take Epsom salts. Also, alkali salts (a mixture of two parts sodium bicarbonate to one part potassium bicarbonate: one teaspoonful in a few ounces of lukewarm water) should help. Discontinue further tests until symptoms have abated once more.

Using this method, you should be able to test one food a day, minimum. Go rapidly if all is well, because the longer you stay off a food, the more the allergy (if there is one) will tend to die down and you may miss it.

Occasionally, patients experience a 'build up' which causes confusion and sometimes failure. Suspect this if you felt better on an exclusion diet, but you gradually became ill again when re-introducing foods, and can't really say why. Perhaps there were no noticeable reactions.

In that case, eliminate all the foods you have re-introduced until your symptoms clear again, then re-introduce them more slowly. This time, eat the foods steadily, several times a day for three to four days before making up your mind. It is unlikely that one will slip the net with this approach.

Once you have accepted a food as safe, of course you must then stop eating it so frequently, otherwise it may become an allergy. Eat it once a day at most — only every four days when you have enough 'safe' foods to accomplish this.

Special instructions for those coming off a fast

Begin only with exotic foods which you don't normally eat. The last thing you want to happen is to get a reaction when beginning to re-introduce foods. Instead, for the first few days, you want to build up a minimum range of 'safe' foods that you can fall back on.

Papaya, rabbit, artichoke and dogfish are the kind of thing to aim for — do the best you can with what is available according to your resources.

The other important point is that you cannot afford the luxury of bringing in one new food a day: you need to go faster than this.

It is possible to test two or even three foods a day when coming off a fast. Pay particular attention to the pulse rate before and after each test meal. It is important to grasp that some symptom, even if not very striking, usually occurs within the first 60 minutes when coming off a fast. You need to be alert to this, or you will miss items and fail to improve without understanding why.

If the worst happens and you are ill by the end of the day and can't say why, condemn all that day's new foods.

The build up of foods is cumulative: that is, you start with Food A. If it is OK then the next meal is Food A + Food B, then A + B + C and so on.

All safe foods are kept up after an allergic reaction. Therefore, if Food F causes a symptom, while you are waiting for it to clear up, you can go on eating foods A-E.

Within a few days, you should have plenty to eat, albeit monotonous. From then on, you can proceed as for those on elimination diets if you wish.

Food diary

It is a good idea to keep a food diary during your experiments with food. Write down everything you eat at each meal and also mark in any symptoms which you experience. It is often possible to spot a pattern which recurs time and time again but which is not evident when only viewing events on a meal-by-meal basis.

It does tend to make you introverted and very conscious of food, which is probably a good thing in the short term. However, taking the long view, it is best not to become too introverted. Eating can become a psychological burden if you go too far. The food diary is merely a tool, not a way of life and should be discontinued as soon as practicable.

CHAPTER 4

Special situations in relation to structured dieting

Apart from the difficulty (and sloth) in changing habits of a lifetime, there are remarkably few problems with exclusion diets. However, one or two situations are worthy of individual comment.

Further exclusion diets

If the simple exclusion diet has not worked for you — or even if it has — you might like to consider alternative eliminations.

For example, you could try following a meat-free diet. Some people do feel better as vegetarians, certainly; but probably more feel ill, however, because of the high incidence of grain and dairy allergies, which are staple foods for vegetarians. Much propaganda is talked about the chemicals present in meat produce. In fact, the chemicals sprayed onto commercial vegetables and fruit constitute a far greater hazard. At least when eating meat you have the animal's liver, which detoxifies chemicals, between you and the poison!

A very useful exclusion diet is the nut- and pip-free diet. This is a wide group of foods and includes several common allergens. Some members of this group come as a surprise: for example, coffee is a nut!

Because such a large number of foods are excluded, it is recommended that you don't go onto the nut- and pip-free diet until you have re-introduced a number of alternatives, perhaps rice or rye or millet, if these are safe. Otherwise you may find yourself with very little to eat.

The full diet is given in Box 12. Follow it for at least one week, longer if you can manage. Then begin challenge testing.

BOX 12

Nut- and pip-free diet

The following foods must be strictly avoided:

Tomatoes, sauce, purées
Apples, pears, plums, damsons, cherries, apricots, peaches
Strawberries, raspberries, gooseberries, blackcurrants
Oranges, lemons, other citrus fruits, marmalade and all fruit juices, squash, fruit flavoured drinks
All varieties of fizzy drinks, including cola
Jellies, instant puddings
Chocolate, cocoa, coffee, and coffee 'creamers'
Grapes, sultanas, raisins, currants, prunes, figs, dates
Nuts, coconut, marzipan, macaroons
Peas, beans, lentils, soya, peanuts
Melon, cucumber, marrow
Spices, pepper, mustard, curry
Cooking oils of all kinds and soft margarines
All herbs (including mint)
Bananas, pineapple

Gluten-free diet

One of the few food allergies accepted by conventionally minded doctors is hypersensitivity to gluten. It is sometimes, but not always, possible to demonstrate antibodies to gluten.

The bowel damage caused by this allergy was eventually discovered to be the cause of coeliac disease, a pernicious wasting illness leading to malnutrition. The patient literally starves while eating normally, because he or she cannot absorb the food being swallowed.

Apart from this very special case, I think gluten allergy is very overrated. A lot of people who get well on a gluten-free diet do so because they are wheat allergic. They can eat rye, oats or barley (the only other foods which contain significant amounts of gluten) with impunity, so gluten cannot be the offender.

Furthermore, other food allergies can cause bowel damage. A diet of raw peas and beans stripped the intestinal lining of experimental rats, exactly as gluten did. In humans, there is often evidence of malabsorption in those with chronic allergic illness where non-gluten dietary factors are to blame.

Try a gluten-free diet if you are suspicious, but you must be prepared to stick to it for a minimum of six to eight weeks to feel any benefit.

Dermatitis herpetiformis, a widespread skin rash with tiny intensely itchy blisters, is said to be associated with gluten sensitivity. Be alert to the possibility if you have this symptom.

For most people the problems of exclusion diets are few. Withdrawal symptoms, extra expense or the sloth encountered in changing the habits of a lifetime, are the main difficulties. However, certain situations require extra comment. These and other matters incidental to dieting are examined below.

Children

There are special considerations when it comes to dieting children, and a compassionate, sympathetic approach is vital.

Probably the biggest barrier to success is that everyone wants to be 'nice' to youngsters, often by feeding them sweets and other junk foods. Even if you are resolved and careful, you will find others ready to break your instructions, albeit behind your back.

Oddly, the best ally is often the child who, once he or she has understood what you are doing, will often refuse treats. It helps to secure the right sort of motivation if you offer some kind of reward. If, in the child's mind, the inducement is worth the effort, then he or she will co-operate with you all the way.

School meals are impossible on any kind of exclusion diet. Either bring the child home, or provide a packed luncheon. Naturally, this cannot be based on sandwiches as is usually the case. Instead, provide a tuck-box with fruit, cold meat cuts and chopped salad. Fruit juice must take the place of squashes, colas and other convenient drinks.

It is best if the challenge tests are done at home when you can personally observe the child. This often limits testing to weekends or school holidays and careful planning is sometimes required.

Remember that withdrawal symptoms can happen with a child also. Be very tolerant for the first few days. He or she may crave favourite foods: just say 'No' and offer an alternative. Eventually, hunger will be on your side.

It's remarkable to watch how a youngster who is a faddy eater (a reliable sign of food allergy) suddenly finds his or her appetite and begins to eat heartily. Perhaps this isn't so surprising; after all, a food allergy is rather like being poisoned — you don't feel like eating much. Also, you will recall the connection between allergy and addiction, which is another reason for strange, unbalanced diets.

I usually advise parents to go on the exclusion diet with the child — for real, and not just in front of him or her. This gives the parents a first-hand idea of what it is like and helps to foster the right sort of attitude. Siblings should also be put on the diet to prevent jealousy or friction. There is an added bonus when the parents or siblings also experience an improvement in health. This happens more often than not, because allergic children come, usually, from allergic families. It is rare, indeed, to have an isolated child with allergies.

Diabetes

The suggestion that diabetes can be a food allergy illness comes as a shock to most people, but this is certainly sometimes the case. I have even got patients successfully off their insulin — something approaching a miracle if the conventional theory about the causation of diabetes is accepted without scrutiny.

For patients managed by drugs and diet alone, there should be little problem. Those on insulin must be very careful about embarking on a low-carbohydrate diet and should not do so without medical supervision.

The simplest modification of the diet is to eat rice as a source of carbohydrate. Better, if you can get help, is systematically to cut down your insulin and reduce your carbohydrate intake by stages. This is always successful, since the accepted practice is to put diabetics on high doses of insulin and then feed them extra carbohydrates! If they didn't take the insulin, they wouldn't need the carbohydrates, and vice versa.

The best challenge test to perform, if you have a glucometer, is to monitor which foods increase your blood glucose, but if not, just carry out the challenge tests in the normal way.

Long-term eliminations

Hopefully, you have now discovered that avoiding certain foods brings about a significant improvement in your health. The long-term implications of this need to be discussed.

Of course, you must avoid the guilty food, at least for a considerable period, though not necessarily indefinitely. It may seem obvious to state this, but I am constantly amazed at the small percentage of patients who, given that they feel better avoiding a food, still can't wait to go back to eating it.

Remember what I said about fixed and variable allergies: that means that, in all probability, you will eventually be able to eat the food again safely, when you have 'rested' it sufficiently.

How long must you stay off the food? This question is rather like, 'How long is a piece of string?' It's an individual variable, but to give you some idea, stay off the food for six months in the first instance. If it still reacts when you give it a proper challenge test, leave it a further twelve months and then repeat the test. If it still reacts, then my advice is, don't bother to try it again.

Beware of sneaking a food back into your diet by taking tiny amounts at first, not enough to make trouble, and then gradually increasing the quantity. This kind of self-deception will only land you back where you started — sick.

Factually, most foods are simple to omit or replace. The main problem is a social one when it comes to items like wheat, sugar, milk and yeast. So much of our day-to-day food contains these substances that it becomes almost impossible to eat out at a restaurant or dine with friends, while still avoiding them. It is certainly getting easier, but until everyone is very much more enlightened it is a problem you will have to face. Just do the best you can without isolating yourself and appearing to be a freak to your friends and family.

Some substitute foods are well known. If cows' milk has to be avoided, goats' milk or sheep's milk products may be suitable, but do test them first. Contrary to the myth, goats' milk does not have medicinal properties. It gets people well by getting them off cows' milk — the real cause of the trouble! (Note: even evaporated milk can be tolerated by some dairy-allergics. Heating it changes its chemical nature and this may be enough to render it safe — but do *test* it first.)

If wheat is a problem, try flours made from rye, barley, rice or millet. If you find that all the grains give you problems, there are still non-cereal flours, such as buckwheat (in the rhubarb family), soya, pea, potato, sago and chestnut flours. Quinoa, a South American plant, is showing considerable promise as a grain substitute for allergics. It should gradually become more readily available.

The main snag is that wheat has an almost unique stickiness that helps to bind in cooking. That is why wheat is so popular. The other gluten grains share it to some extent, but the remainder will simply crumble, so bread is quite impracticable. However, you can make cakes, biscuits and scones using other binders. Egg is best, if you can tolerate it. If not, honey or sugar will stick to some extent. There are egg replacers available such as Bipro (milk-based). Soya flour also helps to stick. Gram flour (chick-pea) is even better, if you can get it.

If all else fails, eat your starch as a mush made with water or fruit juice (like porridge).

For further culinary advice, refer to the available cook books for allergics (see Further Reading).

Adequate nutrition

It is very important not to remain on a long-term diet which is nutritionally inadequate. You will complicate your health problems considerably. If you find yourself reacting badly to a large number of substances, a rotation diet is better.

It is rare indeed to have to avoid completely more than a handful of foods. Usually it is possible to eat even poorly tolerated food on an infrequent basis. *Keep a large repertoire of foods at all times.*

One of the saddest things I see is a patient who has suspected a reaction with food after food and gradually left each out of the diet, until only two or three 'safe' foods are left. This is the high road to disaster. A life of tea, lettuce and toast (a true example) or similar is what lies at the end.

This is not to say that there are not a number of unlucky people who develop many complex reactions to food. The important point is that such reactions, in the main, are not permanent. A correctly constructed rotation diet is the proper answer.

The rotation principle

It is an unfortunate and inconvenient fact that some people develop new allergies very quickly. All it takes is a too frequent exposure to a food or other agent and the trouble starts up.

This can be very annoying. You might work out a safe diet, feel very well for a time and then begin to get your symptoms returning because of this problem. The way to prevent it happening is to ensure that you eat each food only once every few days. We call this the rotation principle.

Luckily, not everyone has to go the whole hog and rotate everything. Nevertheless, it is a good principle to apply and, even if you continue to feel well while excluding one or two foods, it is still a good idea to make sure that you eat the remainder in as varied a manner as possible. At all costs, try to avoid a routine of having just a few foods that you eat over and over again. Make yourself experiment with the new tastes and start to be adventurous with recipes and menus.

The minimum rotation period is four days. Less than that just isn't long enough to rest the food adequately. Some patients feel better rotating one day in five. Very sick patients sometimes can only allow themselves to eat one food per meal, once every seven days, but this is extreme.

You can construct your own rotation diet: a different meat for each day, a different fruit, a different drink and so on. (To do it

---

━━━━━━ *BOX 13* ━━━━━━

Correct rotation of allowed foods

The rule is:

Same food every four days; same family every second day.

DAY	1	2	3	4	1 etc.	
FOOD	wheat	oats	—	barley	wheat	WRONG
FOOD	wheat	—	wheat	—	oats	WRONG
FOOD	wheat	—	oats	—	wheat	CORRECT

━━ *BOX 14* ━━

Seven-day rotation diet

Use fresh foods wherever possible, not tinned or frozen.

DAY	Sunday	Monday	Tuesday
MEAT AND FISH	Halibut Duck Plaice Deer Turkey Anchovy	Chicken Eggs Pheasant Quail Rabbit	Beef Veal Milk Cream Cheese Yogurt Tuna Mackerel Skipjack
VEGETABLES	Peas Beans Liquorice	Cauliflower Swede Brussels sprouts Broccoli	Onions Mushrooms Leek Chanterelle Garlic Yeast Chives Asparagus
FRUIT	Cherry Loganberry Plum Blackberry Peach Strawberry Apricot Raspberry Prunes Grapefruit Lychee	Pineapple Banana	Guava Kiwi fruit
NUTS	Peanuts (Bean family)	Pistachio (Mango family)	Walnut Pecan
GRAIN	Sugar cane	Rye	Wheat
JUICE/DRINK	Grapefruit juice	Pineapple juice	Milk
OIL	Peanut oil	Safflower oil	Soya oil

BOX 14

Seven-day rotation diet (cont)

Use fresh food wherever possible, not tinned or frozen.

Wednesday	Thursday	Friday	Saturday
Pork Ham Bacon Sausage Lard	Cod Salmon Haddock Trout Ling Hake	Herring Pilchard Sardine	Lamb Crab Mutton Lobster Goat Prawn Shrimp
Carrot Celery Parsley Parsnip	Potato Tomato Red, green, yellow pepper Aubergine	Courgette Marrow Spinach Cucumber Pumpkin Olive Sesame	Cabbage Turnip Radish Chinese leaves
Grape Raisin Mango Sultana	Orange Lemon Lime Satsuma	Apple Melon Pear Quince	Rhubarb Papaya Buckwheat Currant Gooseberry

Cashew
   (Mango family)
	Brazil	Almond
		   (Apple family)
			Hazelnut
			Coconut

Oats	Millet Bamboo Barley	Rice	Corn
Grape juice	Orange juice	Apple juice	Blackcurrant juice
Grapeseed oil	Sunflower oil	Sesame oil Olive oil	Rapeseed oil Corn oil

BOX 15

Food family table

The following table gives common foods and their families. No attempt is made here to list all foods or to include all biological families.

PLANT FAMILIES

Fungi or moulds: Baker's yeast (hence breads and doughs, etc.), brewer's yeast (hence alcoholic beverages), mushroom, truffle, chanterelle, cheese, vinegar (hence pickles and sauces)

Grasses: Wheat, corn, barley, oats, millet, cane sugar, bamboo shoots, rice, rye (note that buckwheat is *not* a member of the grass family)

Lily: Onion, asparagus, chives, leek, garlic, sarsaparilla, shallot

Mustard: Broccoli, cabbage, cauliflower, Brussels sprouts, horseradish, kohlrabi, radish, swede, turnip, watercress, mustard and cress

Rose: Apple, pear, quince, almond, apricot, cherry, peach, plum, sloe, blackberry, loganberry, raspberry, strawberry

Pulses or legumes: Pea, chick pea, soya bean (hence TVP), lentils, liquorice, peanut, kidney bean, string bean, haricot bean, mung bean, alfalfa

Citrus: Orange, lemon, grapefruit, tangerine, clementine, ugly, satsuma, lime

Cashew: Cashew nut, mango, pistachio (also poison ivy)

Grape: Wine, champagne, brandy, sherry, raisin, currant, sultana, cream of tartar

Parsley: Carrot, parsley, dill, celery, fennel, parsnip, aniseed

Nightshade: Potato, tomato, tobacco, aubergine, pepper (chilli, paprika)

Gourd: Honeydew melon, watermelon, cucumber, squashes, cantaloup, gherkin, courgette, pumpkin

BOX 15

Food family table (cont)

Composite: Lettuce, chicory, sunflower, safflower, burdock, dandelion, camomile, artichoke, pyrethrum

Mint: Mint, basil, marjoram, oregano, sage, rosemary, thyme

Palm: Coconut, date, sago

Walnut: Walnut, pecan

Goosefoot: Spinach, chard, sugar beet

Sterculia: Chocolate (cacao bean), cocoa, cola nut

The following commonly eaten plants have no *commonly* eaten relatives: juniper, pineapple, yam, banana, vanilla (often a chemical imitation), black pepper, hazelnut, chestnut, fig, avocado, maple, lychee, kiwi fruit, tea, coffee, papaya, brazil nut, ginseng, olive, sweet potato, sesame (also as tahini).

ANIMAL FOOD FAMILIES

Bovines: Cattle (beef), milk and dairy products, mutton, lamb, goat

Poultry: Chicken, eggs, pheasant, quail (*not* turkey)

Duck: Duck, goose

Swine: Pork, bacon, lard (dripping), ham, sausage, pork scratchings

Flatfish: Dab, flounder, halibut, turbot, sole, plaice

Salmon: Salmon, trout

Mackerel: Tuna, bonito, tunny, mackerel, skipjack

Codfish: Haddock, cod, ling (saith), coley, hake

Herring: Pilchard, sardine, herring, rollmop

Molluscs: Snail, abalone, squid, clam, mussel, oyster, scallop

Crustaceans: Lobster, prawn, shrimp, crab, crayfish

The following commonly eaten animals and fishes have no *commonly* eaten relatives: anchovy, sturgeon (caviar), white-fish, turkey, rabbit, deer (venison)

properly you need to know about food families — see Box 15.)

The rules are quite simple. Any single food is allowed every four days. Members of the same food family can appear every second day. Box 13 should make this clear.

A vexed question is whether you should eat a food more than once on the allowed day. Again the answer has to be — try it for yourself and see. Some people can get away with it, some can't.

Sometimes, rotation dieting will show up an allergy by unmasking it. If you start to react on a particular day, test those foods individually (if you wake with the symptoms, of course, you will need to test the previous day's foods).

Pin up a chart of your rotation diet in the kitchen or on the refrigerator door. That will serve as a reminder.

Basically, rotation diets are an onerous chore. Do not follow one unless there is a real need because of the seriousness of your illness or the tendency to develop new allergies.

Finally, I close this section with an example of a seven-day rotation diet drawn up by one of my patients (see Box 14).

Food families

The table in Box 15 gives a list of food families and also foods without commonly eaten relatives. Use this as a guide in making up your own rotation diet.

There is a great deal of cross-reacting between different members of a family. However, this does not mean that if you are allergic to one food all other members of that family are condemned. For example, it is possible to be violently allergic to potato but OK with tomato. It *does* mean that you should be more suspicious.

Note that ham and bacon belong with pork, dairy produce with beef, and eggs with chicken. These actually come from the same animal. Once again, though, it doesn't follow automatically that you will be allergic to both. It is possible to be very allergic to milk and dairy produce and yet (reasonably) safe with beef.

Study the table carefully. It will repay the effort.

CHAPTER 5

Environmental allergies

You may have carried out the dietary elimination and challenge steps diligently and yet feel no better. However, this does not prove you don't have a food allergy. It may mean simply that some other cause of trouble is present at the same time. Some readers may even have discovered they react quite strongly to certain foods, yet recovery remains elusive. The answer could be an allergy to something in the environment.

Something in the air?

Environmental or inhalant allergies are quite common. Indeed, for half a century they were the only kind to be recognized. Allergens can include such diverse substances as pollen, dust-mite (an almost invisible small animal), feathers, mould, fur and fabrics. The one thing these substances all have in common is that they are light enough to float in air and so be breathed in.

Actually, there is an interesting overlap here. Sometimes a food allergic individual may react to food 'dust', that is, inhaled small particles of food. This may happen with flour, during baking, for example!

In addition, we are now beginning to recognize an insidious and potentially more dangerous inhalant problem: chemicals. As atmospheric pollution rises higher and higher, our bodies are subjected to an ever-increasing barrage of toxic substances. Every year in Europe, 25 million tons of sulphur dioxide are released into the air, creating so-called acid rain. This acid rain is said to have eroded 4 per cent of the weight of the city of Dortmund in West Germany; St Paul's cathedral in London has lost 1″ (2.5cm) of its surface in places. If it can do this to solid brick and stone, only a fool would feel that it is safe for humans to breathe, in the long term.

The cheerful fact remains, however, that many people with environmental allergies get well by eliminating foods alone. To understand why this is so, we need to consider a very important bio-medical concept. It is the key to overcoming all disease processes, and should be burned in letters of fire into the brain of every doctor. Unfortunately, it is not even mentioned during training. It is the principle of TOTAL BODY LOAD.

Total body burden

As stated in Chapter 1, the body has a number of wonderful defence mechanisms that work for us. The immune system is only one of these. Others include the roving white blood cells, which eat invading germs, and that stupendous science-laboratory workshop for detoxifying poisons — the liver.

These and other systems operate in harmony to keep us from harm — in fact, certain death — because it is a very hostile world outside our skins. It is only when the defences are overworked that we actually get any problems at all. Every day, every minute, trouble is nipped in the bud before it even gets started.

Thus you will see that a symptom, any symptom, is really quite serious. It means that the defences have already run out. They can no longer cope.

Overloading the system is thus asking for trouble. Allergies are just one way of overloading; chemical toxins are another; drugs themselves, used to treat illness, can be quite toxic and likewise become a burden on the body's resources; add to that tobacco addiction, alcohol, fatigue, poor nutrition (vitamin and mineral deficiencies) and mental stress and you will see our bodies are under a lot of duress. Too much all at one time, and a breakdown is inevitable; we become ill. For some people this means a flare-up of their allergic condition. When you are feeling particularly despondent, you might reflect that this illness is preferable to heart disease or cancer.

The important point is that if you reduce the load by removing *any* one offender, it helps. Thus by eliminating certain key food allergens, you may bring the total burden back to the point where the body can manage; symptoms will subside, *even in the presence of other adverse health factors* (e.g. the person may still be under the same mental stress or still breathing the same toxic chemical, yet he or she returns to feeling well). Sometimes, simple avoidance of one particular food will have this beneficial effect, though admittedly rarely. The result looks almost miraculous.

In actual fact, once you understand the principle, the implications are many and varied. For example, you might find you can eat an allergic food on holiday (where the mental stress and, probably, chemical pollution is far less) but at home it will cause symptoms; if you give up using hairsprays and perfumes your stuffy nose and catarrh may improve, even though dust is the main cause; if you are under stress, you need to eat a safer diet; if you get rid of infections in the body (see Chapter 8) and take vitamin and mineral supplements, you will improve your tolerance of food allergens and so on.

Thus you will see at once this is a very important biological principle and if you understand it and *apply it*, it will serve you well.

Dust and dust-mite

We put these two together for practical purposes; they are probably the most widely known (and suffered) inhalant allergies. Individuals sensitive to one, usually also react badly to the other.

House dust is a mixture of particles of food, human skin scales, hair and grits but the main ingredient is fabric fibres worn from carpets, clothes, upholstery and drapes. House-dust-mite is a living organism and seen under a microscope, looking grotesque and alarming, it seems to well deserve its fearsome scientific name, Dermatophagoides Pterynissinus. Actually the most allergenic part is the excrement. It is found mainly in beds, but also bedroom carpets, bathroom carpets, lounge carpets, loafing chairs and settees — in fact, anywhere that human skin scales fall, since that is what it feeds on.

Rhinitis and asthma are obvious allergy conditions due to dust and dust-mite. What isn't so generally known, however, is that it is often the principal cause of eczema. I am grateful to Dr Paul August for calling this to my attention some years ago. He is a very enlightened dermatologist (skin doctor) and uses the environmental and allergy approach to try and help his patients.

He noted that many eczema patients tend to improve when staying in the Skin Hospital in Manchester and wondered if it wasn't simply that the linen was changed daily, which keeps dust and dust-mite to a minimum. To test this idea, he would get the patient's relatives to bring in dust from the patient's own bedroom and, without saying what he was doing, sprinkle it into the patient's hospital bed while pretending to examine them. If the rash reappeared within 24 hours, he was able presumptively to diagnose a dust allergy!

It is impossible to get rid of dust and dust-mite, but reducing it significantly will help the total body burden. Fighting it is a complicated business, and the best advice I can give is do as much as you can.

The absolute minimum is to lift the bedroom carpet (replace it with lino, tiling or cork) and cover the mattress. It must be a dust-proof or plastic mattress cover. An underblanket can be put over it, then a sheet, but everything outside the cover must be changed and washed at least weekly. It may be necessary more often for cases of severe eczema and asthma.

To go further, remove all sources of dust, such as pelmets, curtains, lampshades, bookshelves and open wardrobes from the bedroom. Vacuum clean it frequently, in all corners, no matter how hard to reach, at least once a week. Ideally, the person who has the allergy should not be present in the room at these cleaning times.

Avoid electric open-bar heaters, convection and especially fan heaters, which all circulate dust. If ducted-air heating is present, it should be blocked off to the room and substituted with a radiator. If there is no central heating, the free-standing oil-filled electric radiators are best (such as the Dimplex model).

Ionizers and air-purifiers (avoid those with scented filters) may help. Try one and see.

Finally, for those allergic to house-dust-mite, there are pesticide sprays available on the market with which to treat the mattress. Those containing methoprene are effective and relatively harmless; the World Health Organization has deemed this substance safe enough to add to drinking water, where there is a risk of infection by mosquito larvae in malarial zones. Be sure the patient doesn't react to aerosol sprays or do it while he or she is absent from the home at least overnight. Follow the instructions exactly. Note, even after using a miticide spray, you must still vacuum the mattress for several more weeks. It is the droppings that cause the reaction and even when no more are being produced, it still takes some time to get rid of all traces. Spray treatment lasts a variable time and needs to be repeated.

Pollens

The cause of hay-fever, pollens, was first discovered by Charles Blackeley in 1873, right here in my own city of Manchester. He sent kites high into the air with sticky plates, saved up pollens and tried sniffing them in winter (he was himself a sufferer) and rubbed samples into his skin to produce what was a very elegant scientific proof.

Hay-fever is characterized by red, itchy eyes, sneezing and catarrh, but any seasonal symptom, made worse by pollens (for example, wheezing and rashes), is covered by the remarks that follow. Certain pollens can be identified because of the time of year when symptoms become manifest. For example, trees begin to pollinate in March and April, grasses in May and June and flowers from June onwards, though there are exceptions to these very broad generalizations. Sometimes the trigger is not a pollen but a seasonal mould.

The main problem is that there is nothing you can do to escape the pollen, or even reduce it, as you can with dust. Short of taking continuous antihistamines, with their tiresome side-effects, or isolating yourself indoors for the best days of the year, the problem has to be tackled some other way.

The secret, once again, is the total body burden. How many people ever think of going on a diet to combat hay-fever?

The logic is simple. If you eliminate any food allergies, the body is better able to cope with inhaled allergies. This is particularly true when it comes to avoiding foods in the grass family, such as wheat, corn, rye, etc., and those with classic hay-fever (grass pollens or hay) are especially benefited. But avoiding milk, food additives, tea, coffee and alcohol can also have a beneficial effect.

It isn't a sure-fire cure, but it is certainly worth a try and anything is better than feeling utterly wretched just when everyone else is having all the fun.

Try the simple elimination diet at a time when the pollen count is high. Even if you don't clear the symptoms, you may reduce your need for medication quite considerably.

Don't forget to follow up the diet with challenge tests, if it works. Find the real culprits. You don't need to stay off the rest.

Best of all, get neutralization therapy from an allergy clinic, if one exists near you. It is safer and more effective than traditional desensitizing injections, which are no longer considered safe (see Chapter 7).

Moulds

Moulds are a serious problem. More food crops worldwide are lost to mould than any other single cause. Yet we need them to rot away rubbish and dead matter. Along with certain bacteria, moulds clean up organic waste and stop the planet becoming a gigantic garbage heap.

Unfortunately, mould allergies are very common. Drug reactions to antibiotics, such as penicillin, are mould allergies. Most exposures, however, come from mould spores floating in the air. Moulds are rather like an all-year-round pollen, only absent during hard frost or when the ground is covered with snow. Suspect mould if you are bad on damp, humid days, but better in cold weather. Also, if damp, musty buildings make you ill, mould is probably the cause.

Different moulds peak at certain times of the year and it may be possible from this to deduce which one is the culprit.

Mould allergy ties in very importantly with the problem of infection with Candida albicans, covered in Chapter 8. Moulds and yeasts are closely related allergenically and a pronounced intolerance to one is usually accompanied by reactions, or cross-reactions, to the other members of the group.

Any symptom can be caused by mould. Stuffy nose is obvious. But the most overlooked symptoms are mental ones. These can be extremely bizarre and frightening. In medieval times people would sometimes eat rye bread infected with ergot mould. This resulted in an intense burning of the skin (St Anthony's fire) and wild, violent and insane behaviour (St Vitus' dance). I have seen patients acting very strangely on mould challenge tests. The trouble is that this distressing manifestation is hardly ever diagnosed because no one ever thinks of it.

Consider mould problems if your house is low-lying in a damp valley (East Lancashire, where the damp valleys favoured the cotton industry, is notoriously bad). Older houses are especially suspect, particularly those with a condensation problem. Sometimes it is possible to see the mould growing on the walls and carpets.

You will need professional advice to be sure of getting rid of the damp. It may entail major structural repairs. If the problem is too extensive, you should consider moving, if you value your health.

In the meantime, a dehumidifier should help to reduce the damp.

Once again, dieting has considerable value. Certain foods are actually moulds (mushrooms and cheese). A suitable diet for a mould-sensitive individual would of course avoid these and also foods containing yeast and fermentation products: alcoholic and fermented drinks, bread (except unleavened), vinegar, sauces, malt and malted foods, yeasted cakes, coffee and chocolate (fermented during processing), B-vitamin products (unless stated yeast-free), over-ripe and mouldy food. Cartoned and bottled fruit juices also contain significant amounts of yeast, but not when freshly squeezed.

Remember that house plants encourage moulds which grow in the damp soil. You may need to get rid of them.

Animal hair and danders

A difficult subject is the question of animals. Allergies to dogs, cats, horses, birds and other pets can cause severe allergies. The obvious solution — get rid of the allergen — is often refused on emotional grounds. People become very attached to their pets.

If you don't think you can bring yourself to undertake the 'logical' solution, you must do the best you can. Certainly removing other allergens will help.

Keep animals out of the bedroom at all costs. That's where you spend the largest segment of the day. Under no circumstances let the pet sleep on the bed. Once fur and dander are present, it can be very difficult to get rid of.

Use the vacuum cleaner often to keep hairs to a minimum.

Beware of your diagnosis. One woman we tested was convinced she was allergic to her horse. It turned out to be a reaction to the dust from the corn feed she was mixing for it!

As with pollens, neutralization therapy may help.

Small rodent urine

The urine of small rodents can be a powerful allergen. This isn't widely known and possibly you have never been told.

I am thinking not so much of rats and mice, but the pets children sometimes keep, such as guinea pigs, hamsters and gerbils. The last two are particularly troublesome since they are often kept in the child's bedroom.

Fortunately, these animals don't live long and pronounced attachments are rare. Don't replace the animal when it dies. Give it away if you can persuade the child. If not, ban it from the bedroom and see that bedding is changed *frequently.*

Chemical allergies

If any one man has established the role that modern chemicals play in the causation of illness, it is Dr Theron Randolph of Chicago. For decades he has argued and demonstrated just how toxic are everyday chemicals that we have been urged, by vested propaganda, to think of as harmless.

It isn't just a question of pesticides and industrial pollution. The two most common chemical allergies I encounter are petrol fumes and house gas. Actually, it isn't correct to call these reactions allergies. It is really low-grade poisoning. Some individuals react at lower doses than others. But the principle is the same and avoidance still the cure.

Another very common offender is formaldehyde, used in many plastics and foams. It is also produced when anything burns, from cigarettes to stoves; plywood, chipboard and laminates give it off; fabrics are treated with it, especially clothes and carpets. There are many more incidences of its use, yet it is very toxic, a strong poison used in fly-sprays and other insecticides. It may even be carcinogenic (the evidence is inconclusive).

Cavity-wall insulation, using urea-formaldehyde foam (UFFI) can contaminate a house for years. It cannot be removed, once installed, and if your problem relates to it, say your symptoms began only after your house was treated, I strongly urge you to move.

There are many other chemical allergies, of course: plastics, urban atmospheric pollution, perfumes and cosmetics, cleaners, solvents, aerosol sprays, paints and food additives, to name but a few. Most of these are derived, ultimately, from petroleum and the whole group we call hydrocarbons. Interestingly, all petroleum (and coal)

BOX 16

Some chemical sources in the home

The following list of chemicals in the home could cause you problems. The list is not exhaustive; there could be others.

Aerosols
Degreasers
Deodorants
Hairsprays
Insecticides

Cleaners
Ammonia
Bleaches
Detergents
Polishes
Soaps

Cosmetics
After-shave
Creams
Deodorants
Perfume
Powders
Talc

Flooring
Carpets
Linoleum
Sealers

Foam rubber
Carpet backing
Cushions
Upholstery

Fuels
Oil
Gas fires
Calor and butane
Coal fires

Leakages
Fridges
Garage (oil)
Heating boilers (flue)

Motor cars
Oil
Petrol
Upholstery

Paints
Oil paints
Paint stripper
Turpentine
Varnish

Solvents
Carbon tetrachloride
Dry-cleaning fluid
Newsprint
Paint stripper

products originated as pine trees in carboniferous forests millions of years ago. Yet we find pine is quite a potent allergen!

Box 16 will give you some idea of the chemicals to look for in your home.

Suspecting chemical allergies

A number of observations should cause you to suspect chemical allergies. You may already be aware that certain substances give you a headache or make you feel sick.

Being made ill by long car journeys is a clue. Also getting a headache due to gloss paint. You may get a rash from a particular cleaning agent. It may even be that certain chemical smells give you a lift! Does that sound silly? Think about glue-sniffers — isn't that exactly what happens to them?

Sometimes the clue is that you are ill in certain places and not in others (this is true with any environmental allergy, not just chemicals). If the city centre makes you tired, sick and headachy, a likely reason is petrol-fume allergy. Patients often tell me they are fine on holiday, either abroad or in the countryside, but when they come back to their city home, they feel ill once again. We can test this out further: we have them return to the city but not go home for the first few hours. If they feel ill at this stage, *before* entering the house, then we know the problem is atmospheric pollution and not allergens within the home. It's a crude test, but worth trying. (See Box 17.)

BOX 17

Symptoms suggesting chemical sensitivity

Bad in enclosed areas (e.g. shopping centres)

Get a lift from or like certain smells

Headache with gloss paint

Loss of smell or heightened smell

React to perfume (ethanol based)

Sick on long car journeys

Unwell in certain locations

Of course the countryside can be a danger zone also, especially during the summer with hazards such as extra pollen, cut grass (hay-making) and, not insignificant these days, chemical pesticide spraying. Almost every week there are newspaper reports of hapless individuals caught inadvertently by crop spraying, some of whom are ill for weeks, even months afterwards. Aircraft are particularly bad in this respect, but tractor spraying can be equally disastrous if the wind is blowing in the wrong direction. When you read these stories, remember we end up eating those exact same crops.

Chemicals at work and school

Don't forget the work environment as a source of chemical exposure. In some trades there are specific hazards and the monitoring of these exposures since the Health and Safety at Work Act of 1974 has come under the control of the Environmental Safety Officer (ESO) in the Environmental Medical Advisory Service (EMAS). However, to pretend this system is working efficiently and protecting workers properly is to be foolish and gullible in the extreme. Only a very small percentage of workers — those employed in larger factories and offices — effectively come under this sort of umbrella.

Although the Act supposedly covers all offices, factories and places of work, in actual fact it is impossible to monitor the countless small businesses that this represents. Only if the individual worker complains is any action likely to be taken in the event of a hazard and many workers are reluctant to report breaches of the codes for fear of losing their jobs, either as retribution or indirectly because the works are closed down due to not being able to afford all the safety procedures required.

It may be obvious to you that you are working with major chemical toxins. Elaborate precautions and safety instructions would tell you that. However, many chemical allergens at work are much more insidious and difficult to detect unless you consider the possibility.

Problems can come from photocopier fluids, solvents, aerosols, powerful cleaning agents and detergents (common where contract cleaners are employed), air purifiers and, last but not least, the fabric of the building and its furnishings (formaldehyde particularly). If your office has that new 'plastic' smell, this could be a problem. Air conditioning often makes matters far worse by circulating indoor pollution.

BOX 18

Symptoms suggesting chemicals at work

Any *known* hazards (e.g. TDI, Formalin)

Better at weekends

Clears up on holidays

Co-workers also affected ('sick building syndrome')

Onset with present employment

Worse Monday-Tuesday

Remember *physical* factors, e.g. VDUs and back or eye strain — not necessarily an allergy.

This problem can be so bad that we have begun to pinpoint what is called the Sick Building Syndrome. Some modern buildings have such a high internal accumulation of these obnoxious substances, that almost everyone feels ill to some degree. Headaches, sore eyes and runny nose, fatigue and inability to concentrate are almost the norm. The effect on work efficiency is disastrous and absenteeism runs sky-high.

Since it is costing industry money in lost man-hours, you may be sure (especially if you are cynical, like me) that a lot of money is now being spent on researching this problem.

In the meantime, the answer is simple. Open the windows! The problem is made far worse by the modern craze for energy efficiency. For allergy sufferers at least, draughts are good news. They help to circulate air and keep down internal pollution. This applies in the home also — double glazing and draught-proofing may be disastrous to those who suffer within the home environment.

The list in Box 18 gives pointers towards allergies in the work environment.

Cleaning up your chemical environment

It makes good sense to clear your environment of as many unnecessary chemicals as possible. This will reduce your overall burden. We choose the home for this because it is something you can control to a great extent. You can't do much about what is beyond your doors and windows (except move if you are downwind from a factory or such) but, unless you have a particularly unsympathetic and selfish family, you should be able to effect enough changes indoors to produce a worthwhile improvement.

Some substances you will be able to replace with safer substitutes. Many you will be able to dispense with altogether. Some you will need and no substitutes can be found. The answer is to recognize the danger, use them as infrequently as possible, preferably get someone else to carry out the task involved and store these substances outside the house, for instance in the garage.

I usually get patients to comb the whole house, room by room, cupboard by cupboard and shelf by shelf, listing all the chemicals found. Sometimes, the list itself is a shock and this is salutary. To pinpoint all potential trouble, I get them to supplement what can be seen with what can be smelled. Most chemical allergics have a very sensitive sense of smell; others have none and will need to enlist the help of someone else. I call this a nose survey: if you can smell it, it can make you ill. That is, if there is enough to cause an odour, there is enough to cause symptoms.

The list of potential chemical allergens shown in Box 16 will help you search out trouble. Store, replace or throw out as much as possible of what you find.

Don't forget carpets and upholstery are potential hazards. Nowadays, most are treated with complex stain-repellent and preservative chemicals. You may not want to throw out your nice new carpet or sofa but at least if you can diagnose that's where the trouble is coming from, you will feel less distressed. Things will probably improve in time. However, for an unlucky few, the truth is simple, if bleak: they will never be well until the luxury wall-to-wall hazard is disposed of!

Organic foods

It pays to avoid food additives and eat only wholefoods, although it must be said there is some hysteria about 'E numbers' at present. Only a very small percentage of the population can never eat foods containing them. For the rest of us, it is a matter of prudence and need not be magnified to become a fear of poisoning.

Probably the greatest hazard is from chemicals sprayed on our foods before harvesting. This can include fertilizers, weedkillers, insecticides, fungicides and others. According to official figures, 98 per cent of green leaf crops, 94 per cent of orchard crops and 95 per cent of root crops are treated with chemicals. Sometimes foods are sprayed after gathering, to assist in storing. All of this poses a serious long-term health threat that has not been properly evaluated.

Foods grown without such chemicals are christened 'organic' or 'organically grown' and developments in this area are a welcome, fast growing trend. Those with serious chemical allergies are advised to eat only organically grown food. However, it is difficult to get supplies and, fortunately, most people don't need to be strict in this regard.

A few weeks' experimentation with elimination and carefully judged challenge tests, comparing organic with non-organic ordinary commercial supplies, should settle the matter.

For years, we have recommended a company called Foodwatch Ltd. Henry Doubleday Research Association Ltd publishes a book listing organic food suppliers, but it suffers from going out of date too quickly. Finally, Action Against Allergy will usually be able to supply names and addresses of organic food suppliers and other chemical-free or allergy-safe household goods. Details of these and other useful addresses are given at the end of the book.

CHAPTER 6

Nutrition against allergies

It is wrong to think of allergies in isolation. We're considering the whole body here (a holistic approach) and allergy is unlikely to be the only malfunction when a person is sick, just as it is unlikely that a headache exists without an underlying cause.

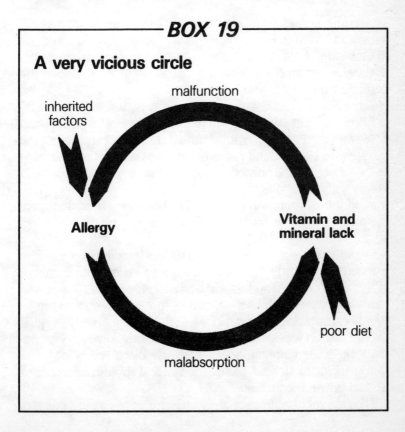

─── BOX 19 ───

A very vicious circle

inherited factors

malfunction

Allergy

Vitamin and mineral lack

malabsorption

poor diet

One of the commonest concomitants of allergy is vitamin and mineral imbalance. This can be directly due to a faulty diet — the modern, so-called balanced diet is often a nutritional disaster — or indirectly, as a result of a failure of the bowel lining to absorb nutrients adequately.

Attention to this fact is important because lack of certain essential nutrients actually seems to predispose to allergy and will make matters worse if unremedied. It can become a self-perpetuating situation, lack of one causing the other, and vice versa (see Box 19). We always break this vicious circle by eliminating allergies. But it makes sense to move on as soon as possible to supplementing vitamins and minerals intelligently.

Vitamins

The name comes from *vital amines*. It was found that these substances were essential for health and yet our bodies could not manufacture them. If there is not sufficient in our food, we suffer disease. For example, a lack of adequate vitamin B_1 causes the condition beri-beri.

Some vitamins have names, for example B_1 is thiamine and B_2 is riboflavin, but eventually a letter coding system was adopted. This started off all right, with vitamins A, B, C, D and E, but the next few were later found not to be vitamins and so there are gaps in the sequence. The only other one that now remains is K. Possibly others will come to light.

In addition, vitamin B was found to be a complicated mixture of substances and so this was subdivided; B_1, B_2, etc. B_4 is missing, so are 7-11, but we have a B_{12}.

You will hear many other vitamin names bandied about. We've reached B_{17}, according to some enthusiasts. Please note that these labels are not official and should be discontinued until it is proved that a substance truly is a vitamin — that is, essential to life.

Other substances important for health, and apparently working in conjunction with vitamins, we call co-factors. Some are vitamin-like, others are simply minerals (these are discussed below). Co-factors include folic acid, biotin, inositol and choline, all reckoned as part of the B complex.

The amount of vitamin or co-factor required to do the job is very

small, but here we immediately get into controversy. The official
view is that there can be tables listing what are called recommended
dietary allowances (RDAs) of vitamins, but the validity of such
figures is questionable, to say the least.

To begin with, the amounts quoted for the United Kingdom are
based on what it takes to avoid diseases like pellagra (B_6 deficiency)
and scurvy (vitamin C deficiency), *not* what it takes for optimum
health. Secondly, such figures make no allowance for the alteration
in requirements in a given individual. In times of stress or disease,
the requirements for individual vitamins may rise enormously.

Last, but not least, it ignores the second hugely important bio-
medical principle — that of biological variation. Everyone is
different, actually unique. To say that everyone requires the same
amount of a vitamin is as stupid as saying we all have blonde hair
and blue eyes — it simply isn't true. One individual may find it
impossible to remain healthy on ten times the dose that keeps
another well.

Remember that what a person eats in his diet may bear no relation
to the amount he actually absorbs. If the bowel isn't performing
adequately, as I have implied might be the case, he might very well
be passing most of the nutrients in his diet straight through in his
faeces.

The myth of the 'balanced diet' also needs debunking. Because
of processing methods, modern foods are sadly depleted in essential
vitamins and minerals. The term 'balanced rubbish' would
communicate more accurately. Eating wholefood is rather better
but even then, with technological, aggressive farming methods,
plants are often forced so fast and to such inflated yields, that they
haven't time to grow as Nature intended and enrich themselves
properly with nutrient goodness from Mother Earth.

An even more ominous recent trend is that of irradiating fruits
to stop them rotting. I'm not concerned with the nuclear radiation
safety factor in this — that seems the least likely hazard. What
I do object to is that foods can now be kept 'fresh' for many
weeks past their usual shelflife. In this time, the vitamin content
steadily declines and after a while the food becomes useless as
a supply of nutrients, even though it may still look shiny and
crisp.

Finally, most modern 'processing' removes the bulk of nutrient
goodness from foodstuffs. What reaches the packet or tin is often

no more than a reconstituted travesty of the food it once was, minus vitamins and minerals.

Still believe in the 'balanced diet'? Dismiss the idea that we are well fed. While it is true we don't have the malnutrition of former times, the evidence of vitamin deficiency is all around in Western society, if you only know what to look for. The trouble is, few doctors do!

Minerals

A number of mineral substances are vital for health. For example, it has long been known that lack of iron leads to anaemia and iodine deficiency gives rise to goitre and loss of thyroid function.

In fact, in recent years, there has been a huge expansion in our understanding of minerals and the part they play in our metabolism. You are referred to fuller texts on this topic, if you are interested, but just to give you an idea of the diverse ramifications of mineral deficiencies, I have selected a few particulars that should whet your curiosity.

Probably the most important element to be studied in recent years is zinc. It has been found to be important in preventing dwarfism, infertility, hair loss, poor skin, diarrhoea, bad wound healing, immune deficiencies and anorexia nervosa. Selenium is important for the elasticity of tissues and so helps to prevent ageing. It may even be important in the defence against cancer. Chromium is important in carbohydrate metabolism and lack of it may predispose to diabetes. We call these substances trace elements because the amounts needed are very small. It is probable that in years to come other essential trace elements will emerge.

Essential fatty acids (EFAs)

Almost accorded the status of vitamins are certain essential fatty acids (EFAs). The body cannot make them but they are vital for optimum health. Chief among these is linolenic acid, found in oil of evening primrose, safflower oil and, to a lesser extent, sunflower and other cold-pressed seed oil extracts.

Linolenic acid is a precursor of prostaglandin E_1, an active metabolite which has a number of valuable properties. It seems to inhibit inflammation, which can be very important to conditions such as rheumatoid arthritis and eczema. More importantly, it antagonizes prostaglandin E_2 which naturally occurs in the body and causes reddening and pain.

Note that its beneficial effects are dependent upon adequate intake of B_6, zinc, vitamin C and niacin. It is no use supplementing linolenic acid alone, without these and other additional substances.

Probably most people would benefit from extra linolenic acids. Modern processed diets are very deficient in it. But certain allergic conditions are especially helped: eczema, hyperactivity, arthritis, PMT and obesity.

Nutrition and allergies

Nutrition, as you can see, is a complex and rapidly expanding field. Even experts admit there is still much to learn and, meanwhile, our knowledge must remain incomplete and our understanding limited. That does not mean, however, that we should do nothing.

Vitamin and mineral supplements certainly help but it seems sensible, in view of the complexity, to limit ourselves to the evidence that has a bearing on allergies and the optimum functioning of the immune system. To that end, I have extracted the important information and present it below.

Vitamin C
Guinea pigs kept deficient in vitamin C have reduced T-lymphocyte numbers but if given excess vitamin C, lymphocytes increase in numbers.

Vitamin B_2 (Riboflavin)
In the presence of B_2 deficiency, there is decreased antibody production.

Vitamin B_6
Lack of B_6 seems to lead consistently to impaired cellular immune functions and decreased antibody production. The thymus is essential to T-lymphocyte function and this organ shrinks in the absence of B_6

Pantothenic acid
As with B_6, there is loss of thymus tissue. Experimental animals

suffer reduced antibody production when pantothenic acid is deficient.

Folic acid
Deficiency leads to a decrease in resistance and impaired lymphocyte function in both humans and experimental animals.

Vitamin B_{12}
It is very difficult to induce B_{12} deficiency in animals but the few animal studies that have been done suggest it is important for lymphocyte functions.

Vitamin A
Experimental animals lacking vitamin A experience a decrease in the number of circulating lymphocytes and loss of thymus tissue. Surgery patients given 30,000–50,000IU vitamin A daily for seven days prior to surgery did not experience the usual post-operational drop in lymphocyte count.

Vitamin E
Antibodies increase two- to three-fold in experimental animals fed on excess vitamin E. When deficient in this vitamin, no antibodies at all were produced.

Iron
Either excess, or lack of, iron has a profound effect on the immune system.

Zinc
Lack of zinc undoubtedly impairs immune function and reduces the competence of other defence mechanisms. Deficiency also leads to shrinkage of the thymus, spleen, lymph nodes and intestinal lymph nodes, resulting in depletion of all classes of lymphocytes.

Calcium
One of the components of the antigen-antibody binding reaction needs calcium. Lack of it also inhibits the function of lymphocytes.

Magnesium
This is important in many body reactions, including nervous tissue function and cellular defence. Certain cancers related to the immune system appear to increase in experimental animals

lacking magnesium, suggesting it is vital in proper immune functioning.

Selenium
Works with vitamin E and is important in immune functions, being involved somehow in antibody production.

Dosages

It might seem odd suggesting doses after what was said about biological variations and requirements. Nevertheless, some assumptions need to be made.

One method is to take large doses to make sure there is more than enough (few vitamins are toxic). This is called megavitamin therapy, but I don't recommend it. It is wasteful and not certain to be safe. For example, overdosing with vitamin A, D and B_6 can have serious consequences.

A better approach is to try and work out what you need, the so-called orthomolecular approach. The idea is to take increasing doses of each vitamin, until you get as much improvement as seems possible. This isn't easy because the effects are both subtle and long term.

In general, the doses chosen are moderate, but much higher than the RDAs (10–100 times larger). It would be prudent to benefit from others' experience as a guide and so I have listed some suggested amounts (Box 20). Remember this is not a prescription, and for some people, double these doses is about right, short term.

Undoubtedly, the easiest way of taking vitamin and mineral supplements is by means of a well formulated multi-preparation. You can always add extra of individual requirements, if that seems to suit you better.

Do remember that it is possible to react to vitamins. Don't be puzzled if this happens. B vitamins are synthesized from yeast; vitamin E usually comes from wheatgerm; vitamin C from corn and so on.

Always get hypo-allergenic supplies. Those free of unnecessary starches, sugars, colours, etc. are best. However, there is no such thing as a non-allergenic vitamin preparation.

This sort of supplementation should be continued for 3–12 months, depending on the patient's general state of health or

— *BOX 20* —

Table of suggested vitamin and mineral doses

Vitamin B$_1$	25mg
Vitamin B$_2$	25mg
Niacin	50mg
Pantothenic acid	100mg
Vitamin B$_6$	50mg
Vitamin B$_{12}$	50mcg
Folic acid	500mcg
Inositol	250mg
Biotin	300mcg
Choline	250mg
Vitamin A	5000IU
Vitamin E	200IU
Vitamin C	250mg
Vitamin D	500IU
Zinc	15mg
Magnesium	200mg
Manganese	1mg
Chromium	200mcg
Selenium	25mcg
Oil of evening primrose	1500mg

debility. Even when the body is very deficient, it still only absorbs nutrients very slowly and so it is a long-term strategy.

With improved digestion and a good diet, it isn't necessary to take vitamins for life. However, it's something which certain people need to do repeatedly for optimum health.

Special situations benefiting from vitamin and mineral therapy

There are many conditions that would benefit from vitamin and mineral therapy. I have chosen just a few that are relevant to this text.

Chemical reactions

Anyone experiencing an acute reaction to chemicals should try taking vitamin C in large doses. It often helps.

To work out how much vitamin C you can tolerate, take increasing doses, 2g (2,000mg) more each time, until you get diarrhoea. Then cut back. So if 10g gives you diarrhoea, take 8g. Even without diarrhoea you should not take more than about 12g.

Note: this is for special situations, for example a long car journey or when you have inadvertently been exposed to a large dose of chemicals. *Do not under any circumstances take this dose as a daily routine.* It isn't that vitamin C is toxic, but you will find you get the signs of scurvy when you go back to normal, or even above normal, levels.

Premenstrual tension

PMT is helped enormously by the allergy diet approach. Some women find they only need to avoid their trigger foods at, or just before, the time of their period. For the rest of the cycle they can eat and drink most foods.

Certain vitamins and minerals also help. Chief among these is vitamin B_6, but it is found to be far more effective taken with magnesium, zinc and gamma-linolenic acid. Again this regime can be confined to about the time of menstruation or beginning just before PMT symptoms are due to start. Suggested doses:

B_6	100mg
Magnesium	600mg
Zinc	25mg
Oil of evening primrose	3,000mg (6 capsules daily)

Adrenal stress

The adrenal gland is a vital organ which secretes a number of hormones to help combat stress and debility, but at times of chronic sickness, for example with a long-term allergenic disorder, it can seem to get truly exhausted!

Correcting this condition lies with a better life style, less stress, a corrected diet and patience. It takes time, but once again certain vitamins and minerals appear to help. Suggested supplements:

Vitamin B_6	100mg
Pantothenic acid	500mg
Magnesium	400mg
Vitamin C	1,000mg

Children's behavioural disorders

Children's behavioural disorders, so-called hyperkinetic syndrome (hyperactivity) and even teenage vandalism and aggression, can be much improved by the allergy diet approach.

Other factors are many and varied and I do not exclude social factors, genetic disposition and psychological deficiencies. The trouble is that we can't do anything about these factors, so it is not what I would call practical science.

The one remaining area of attack is nutritional supplements. Here there are two clear winners — zinc and gamma-linolenic acid.

Make sure your child has a good vitamin and mineral supplementation (the doses I suggested for adults could be halved or quartered), but be sure to add, daily:

Zinc   15mg
Oil of evening primrose   2-3 capsules

Coming off tranquillizers

We all know that far too many tranquillizers are prescribed. Often the trouble is not anxiety in the first place. What is particularly disturbing is that the patient is often not told that the drug being prescribed is a tranquillizer. They go on taking it in good faith, and then find themselves addicted.

The withdrawal symptoms when coming off tranquillizers can be very severe at times, but these are eased by taking large doses of B vitamins. If you are struggling to get off tranquillizers, and similar drugs, try the following:

Vitamin B_1 100mg
Vitamin B_2 100mg
Pantothenic acid   500mg
Niacin   500mg
Magnesium   600mg
Vitamin B_6 200mg

This is for short-term use only (2-3 weeks). Note: this dose of niacin (nicotinic acid) will produce a skin burning akin to too much sunshine. This unpleasant side-effect is nothing to be alarmed about. Your body will become accustomed to this dose within a few days.

CHAPTER 7

Special testing methods

Most of this book has been devoted to information to help you sort out your own allergy problem, if you are unlucky enough to have to do that. Sometimes, however, it is not possible to solve an allergic illness without expert help. If recovery isn't simple and straightforward, you are advised to contact one of the modern allergy centres, otherwise you could make matters worse by floundering about, doing the wrong things.

There follows a rapid overview of a number of possible testing and treatment methods you may encounter if you find yourself attending a professional. There is such a variety of approaches it can be very difficult for the layman to know what to do for the best. Different centres may use individual methods, some of which seem to be more successful than others or which have a different emphasis. It is hoped that this chapter will help to dispel any confusion.

The holistic approach

In a sense, of course, all treatment is valid allergy treatment. Bearing in mind what I said about total body burden, you will readily see that psychotherapy, an exercise programme, yoga, retirement from work on health grounds, cleaning up incidental infections, osteopathy and even divorce are all actions which will have some bearing on the allergy complaint.

Similarly, acupuncture, homoeopathy and other holistic approaches may very well help, at times even effect a cure.

But these are not what I would call allergy treatments, as such, and for the sake of brevity and comprehensibility, I have narrowed

76 _____The allergy handbook

down my target to those treatments which may be said to be unique to allergies.

I hope that in what follows you will find the relief you are looking for if you have not already found it in the earlier chapters of the book.

Conventional allergy treatments

Conventional allergy detection has not significantly advanced since 1911, when the prick and scratch test method was first developed. A small drop of test reagent is dropped onto the skin which is then scratched or pricked with a needle at that spot. The amount of flare and wheal compared to a control (inert) solution gives an indication of how allergic the substance is.

It is a very inaccurate method, with many false negatives and food hardly reacts at all this way, though a demonstrable allergy may be present on challenge testing. Because it can be misleading, many conventional allergists prefer not to use it.

This method aims to find out which substances the patient was allergic to, then to give injections of a mixture of these, increasing gradually in strength, until quite large amounts were being tolerated. The body was often found then to be able to cope with normal ambient concentrations. This is called desensitization.

There are two drawbacks to this treatment: (a) it rarely works; (b) it is extremely dangerous. Patients sometimes react severely and deaths occur regularly. (Those who are offered treatment are never told this, I find!) So risky is it, in fact, that the advisability of it was debated in the *British Medical Journal* and other medical publications (1986) and the consensus view was that it should be discontinued.

Patch testing

Also fairly primitive in technique is patch testing. Small quantities of different suspected substances are placed under individual patches which are taped to the skin for a number of hours. A reddening of the skin under the patch denotes a sensitivity to that substance. A control is used, since some people react to the pads or tape etc.

A positive reaction is probably fairly dependable but it rarely happens. Even substances known to have a marked effect often don't affect the skin. Negative reactions do *not* exclude significant allergens.

This method works best for identifying causes of contact dermatitis, such as nickel, soap powders or industrial chemicals.

The RAST test

The only other remaining conventional test of note is the radio-allergo-sorbent test (RAST) for antibodies to foods, dusts and other allergens. I do not propose to describe the method, which is complex, technical, and expensive, and, in my view, of little value.

The cytotoxic test

Sometimes celebrities inadvertently promote an allergy approach. James Coburn, the film actor, was incapacitated by arthritis until this method showed he was allergic to a number of common foods and opened the door to a cure. The last I heard, he was as active as any other man his age.

All it takes is a blood sample from the patient. It is centrifuged to allow the white cells to be removed in bulk, which are then tested against a battery of foods, inhalants and common chemicals.

If an allergy to one of these substances exists, the white cells are damaged and finally killed, hence the name: cyto — of a cell. It is then possible to grade the reactions somewhat, which helps to give an idea of the severity of the allergy: 0 = no reactions; 1 = mild; 2 = moderate; 3 = severe.

The method is easy for the patient, it only takes a few minutes to give a blood sample and is relatively cheap.

On the other hand, it isn't entirely accurate (I have seen false negatives inhibit recovery), laboratories tend to give inadequate advice and, most important, they do not make it clear that this test is nothing more than a transient picture of the patient's intolerances. It could be invalid after as little as a few weeks. Almost certainly it will be after a few months.

Yet the patient is left avoiding certain foods indefinitely, with no clear plan in mind, struggling to keep up an adequate diet on a selection of things to eat that may be pitifully limited.

No method is entirely accurate, of course, and successes with the cytotoxic test can be dramatic. Just bear the criticisms in mind.

The main UK Laboratory is listed in Useful Addresses at the end of the book.

Miller's method

(Also known as provocation and neutralization, or serial end-point skin titration)
This is a natural development from the prick or scratch tests. The food, dust or chemical reagent is injected superficially into the skin, making a deliberate wheal. If this grows (compared to a control) over, say, ten minutes, this suggests an allergy. Sometimes a symptom is produced (provocation) and this is much more conclusive. Remember these substances are tested one at a time, so there is no doubt which causes the symptom.

If a reaction occurs, the patient is then given a series of injections, getting *weaker*, at ten-minute intervals, until the wheal ceases to grow and the symptom, if there is one, disappears completely.

This 'switch-off' dilution is called the neutralizing dose and it is a kind of antidote. Usually the patient takes a cocktail of these neutralizing doses, one drop under the tongue just before meals and he or she can then often eat the food without reacting to it. A percentage of patients, however, obtain relief only if they inject the neutralizing mixture — once or twice a week is usually sufficient.

All this can be done blind or double-blind but in ordinary routine work at the clinic this is an unnecessary labour. Most patients, I find, are very reliable observers.

The main advantages to this method are that the symptom gives the patient a vivid subjective demonstration of each troublemaker, which helps to fix them in his or her mind. Also the patient isn't restricted to a very meagre diet; allergic foods can be eaten in moderation, under the umbrella of the 'drops'. Only severe offenders are banned and even these may be desensitized by taking the drops and resting the food for several months.

I like this method best of all and we rely on it heavily at my clinic. But, it must be admitted, there are limitations. Patients with many complex allergies are sometimes not much helped by the neutralizing doses. These are the very people who would most benefit from them.

Sometimes, end-points shift rapidly and may need frequent re-testing, which can be an ongoing expense.

But even if the 'drops' are not effective, this still remains a good diagnostic method and can rapidly pinpoint the worst allergies for a patient.

It is completely safe. This is because we are going *weaker* instead of stronger, as in the now banned conventional densensitization. Reactions are common, but rarely severe, and in any event relieved by finding the corresponding neutralizing dose.

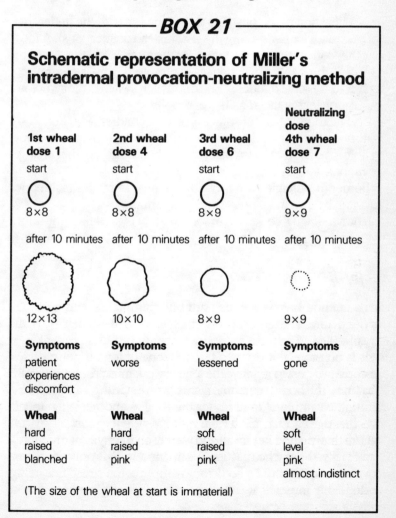

─────── **BOX 21** ───────

Schematic representation of Miller's intradermal provocation-neutralizing method

			Neutralizing dose
1st wheal dose 1	**2nd wheal dose 4**	**3rd wheal dose 6**	**4th wheal dose 7**
start	start	start	start
8×8	8×8	8×9	9×9
after 10 minutes	after 10 minutes	after 10 minutes	after 10 minutes
12×13	10×10	8×9	9×9
Symptoms	**Symptoms**	**Symptoms**	**Symptoms**
patient experiences discomfort	worse	lessened	gone
Wheal	**Wheal**	**Wheal**	**Wheal**
hard	hard	soft	soft
raised	raised	raised	level
blanched	pink	pink	pink
			almost indistinct

(The size of the wheal at start is immaterial)

For the majority of people, then, it is quick, easy and safe, allowing the maximum freedom in choosing dietary items. It works equally well for environmental substances and is a boon for allergies to common substances, such as gas and petrol fumes, which are impossible to avoid.

Sub-lingual provocation and neutralization method

A modification of the previous technique is to use the under-the-tongue route for performing the test (instead of injections). A food or other concentrate is placed under the tongue and the reactions noted. If the patient experiences a symptom, this is neutralized as before, by serial dilutions. The one which switches the symptom off completely is taken as the end-point.

The method is helpful sometimes with children who don't like injections but only if they can describe their symptoms, or some visible reaction occurs (such as unruly behaviour or other change of mood).

Borderline allergies will probably be missed by this technique. Obviously, any that show up are important.

The sub-lingual cocktail used for treatment is essentially the same, whichever titration method is used.

Applied kinesiology

This method has its origins partly in chiropractic and partly in acupuncture. The discovery on which it is based is that if the body is subjected to adverse influences, certain muscles go weak.

It is possible, therefore, to test the tone of a group of muscles (techniques exist to improve the tone of weak muscles and generally 'balance' the body's dynamic status before starting), and then, by putting a sample of food under the tongue and retesting, to tell whether that substance is hostile to the body. If the muscles weaken significantly, the food is deemed to be an allergen.

Actually, those who practise this method say it is only necessary for the patient to hold a bottle or a sample of the substance being tested, the muscles will still go weak. That means non-food substances can be tested also.

This method has the great advantage of being very quick and inexpensive. Thus it would probably suit the overworked GP who has to work within NHS financial constraints.

It probably isn't as accurate as the more 'scientific' methods, but that doesn't mean it isn't successful most of the time. Remember it isn't necessary to get absolutely every allergy to make someone well.

Even if it was only 60–70 per cent accurate (and is probably much better than that when carried out by a skilled practitioner), it is still the most cost-effective method of all.

The Vega machine

Developed in Germany by Dr Schimmel and now increasingly in use in the UK, this strange gadget certainly has an exciting future.

BOX 22

The Vega testing machine

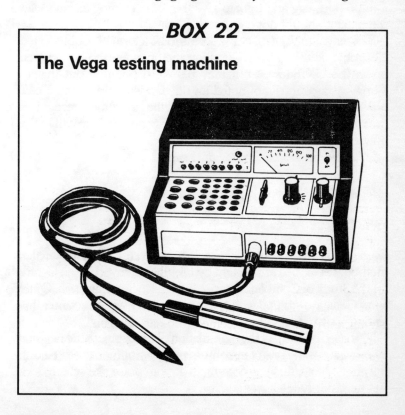

The Vega machine (Box 22) is basically a Wheatstone bridge. The patient holds one electrode in his hand; the other is a probe which the practitioner uses to touch one of numerous critical spots on the body, which produce a read (a swing of the needle). The circuit includes a metallic honeycomb into which different solutions are placed for testing. The machine is calibrated by putting poison, such as a phial of Paraquat, in the honeycomb. This produces a 'disorder' read (a drop in register). The pathogenic potential of any test substance that gives the same read as paraquat should be obvious.

The Vega machine is said to be useful in detecting many conditions, including stressed organs, early cancer, imbalances and even too much electromagnetic radiation from living close to high-tension electric cables.

From the point of view of this text, the important capability of the Vega machine is that it can be used for allergy testing. Obviously, if milk, port, egg and tomato give the same reading as Paraquat, the patient should not eat them!

Basically, the Vega machine seems to be a form of sophisticated electronic dowsing. Such detection methods tend to be frowned on in the UK. However, it may be worth pointing out that in Germany, a country not noted for dilettantism and flighty ideas, dowsers enjoy a much better status. Even the government recognizes the value of dowsing and many doctors are not afraid to call in the dowser on a difficult case.

Is it we who are backward, or they?

The auriculo-cardiac-reflex method (ACR)

Even stranger than applied kinesiology is the auriculo-cardiac-reflex method, developed and taught by Dr Julian Kenyon of the Centre for the Study of Complementary Medicine in Southampton. Quite a few GPs have studied with him and you may well encounter this testing technique.

It is based on the fact that stimulation of the sympathetic nervous system causes the rate of maximum pulse amplitude to shift along the artery. Note: this has nothing to do with pulse rate, which does not necessarily alter.

The test is calibrated as follows: the practitioner rests his thumb over the radial artery at the wrist so that the impulse is just out of reach beyond the tip of his thumb. A bright light is then shone onto a sympathetically enervated portion of skin, either the earlobe or the back of the hand. This causes the point of maximum amplitude of the pulse to move till it comes directly under his thumb. Done properly, it is like feeling nothing until the light shines, at which point the pulse suddenly starts to bump under the counting thumb. This response to light is called a positive reflex.

Testing foods and other allergens is then simply a matter of holding filters containing each substance over the skin of the forearm. A positive auriculo-cardiac reflex lasting a dozen or more pulse-beats is a sign of an allergy. If it lasts 20 or more beats, that is a severe allergy.

With a set of filters covering common foods and allergens, it is possible to test quickly a wide range of substances. Once again, the patient must simply avoid the food but, since only the most pronounced allergens show up, it doesn't usually lead to a long list of banned substances.

As with the applied kinesiology method, the ACR is a fast and cost-effective means of allergy testing, sacrificing high accuracy for expediency but a very useful method, nonetheless.

The total environmental control unit

Until recently, there was no testing unit of this type in Europe but since Dr Jonathan Maberley opened one in Keighley, Yorkshire, this resumé of methods would be incomplete without describing it.

The basic idea is to isolate the patient *completely* from the everyday environment. As well as fasting for five days, he or she is cocooned in a special building with filtered air supply and only special water to drink. Flooring, wall-coverings, curtains, etc. are absent or specially chosen to be chemically inert. No plastics are allowed, bedding and personal linen may only be natural fabrics. By attention to meticulous small details, every care is taken to ensure that the patient is not exposed to unnecessary chemicals. Even the clothing and personal habits of the ancillary staff come under scrutiny, just as in an isolation hospital, except that, instead of trying to prevent pathogens getting out, this is to prevent them getting in!

You will see that this follows the fasting principle but is taking it to its logical conclusion and trying to unmask *all* potential allergens. The body burden is reduced enormously and it is possible to say with some confidence that if the patient doesn't get well in a unit like this, his or her illness is not primarily an allergy or environmental one. This fact alone could have some value.

After the five days of fasting, food challenge tests begin, using only pure organically grown supplies, prepared in a special kitchen to ensure that the food is not contaminated with chemicals, such as North Sea gas, during cooking. This stage may take a week or more.

Finally, the patient can go on to chemical testing, which is done in a special booth where concentrations can be carefully monitored.

After about three weeks of this approach, the patient has had a comprehensive work-up of their food and environmental allergies and should know exactly where they stand. Modifications in his or her home and lifestyle will be necessary but at least these can be done to a plan and not haphazardly.

I've heard it said that the biggest problem with units of this type (there are two already operating in the USA) is trying to re-integrate patients with the everyday world. Going home means being exposed once again to a bombardment of chemical triggers and sometimes this makes the patient very ill before he or she has even had time to modify the home. However, Dr Maberley assures me that, though this is a valid and important theoretical risk, in practice there is surprisingly little trouble.

The biggest real stumbling block is cost: approximately £800 per week at the time of writing.

Enzyme potentiated desensitization (EPD)

A bridge between conventional desensitization and low-dose neutralization is Dr Len McEwen's method of enzyme potentiated densensitization.

It is definitely a vaccine approach, whereas Miller's neutralizing method seems to be more akin to the antidote principle. Briefly, in EPD a cup is taped over the forearm, after scarifying the skin to remove the waterproof layers. Under this cup is placed a vaccine containing dozens of commonly encountered food and environmental substances, along with certain enzymes to make it work (hence the name). The cup is kept in place for 24 hours and then removed.

Antigens soak into the blood over several hours and this creates a favourable antibody response. Obviously not every ingredient will succeed but since there are over 80 foodstuffs, even if only half worked this would mean a significant improvement to many patients.

The doses used are extremely small. In fact more food appears in the blood after eating a meal than from this technique. It is vital therefore that the patient avoid food the day before, the day of and the day after treatment. Two simple foods are used, such as lamb and carrot. Alternatively, a synthetic diet substitute, such as Vivonex or Elemental 08 can be used.

The treatment takes up to twelve months to produce worthwhile improvement for complex food allergies. Environmental allergies, such as grass, pollen and house dust respond much quicker.

McEwen estimates EPD is about 85 per cent successful. It doesn't work for chemical allergies or insect bites.

Dowsing

It seems proper to include more than a passing reference to dowsing because you may meet it. Usually a lock of hair is asked for. Sometimes, the term hair analysis is used, but this should *not* be confused with scientific hair analysis for minerals carried out by reputable laboratories using a mass spectrograph. For one thing, these laboratory tests cannot give any information about allergies or even vitamin status from a hair sample. Dowsers will claim to do this.

Typically, the dowser uses a pendulum which is swung over the hair sample. It gives an altered swing for an allergy.

I have no objection to this sort of thing, provided it is made clear that dowsing is involved (which isn't usually the case). The cost is generally moderate (about £10), so in my view no one is being cheated or robbed. I can certainly point to a number of instances in my files where improvement has taken place by avoiding dowsed foods. In the case of one girl, her dowsed list was very similar to what we found on serial end-point skin titration.

There has been a lot of criticism recently of dowsing for allergies, in the press and on television. The dowsers are partly to blame for giving themselves pseudo-medical authority by calling their centres 'clinics'. Allergy treatments should always be carried out by trained medical staff, otherwise serious illnesses *not* due to allergy may be overlooked and the patient endangered.

Since there are so many methods available you can probably deduce that no one of them is exactly right; each one has its pros and cons. If any one method did everything we want (fast, cheap, accurate and with a therapeutic spin-off), it would long ago have established itself as *the* method to use.

At least you can now approach a clinic or doctor and ask intelligent questions about what methods are used and, hopefully, in that way you may undergo testing that you feel comfortable about and comprehend, at least in outline.

Allergy patients must understand as much as possible about the allergy phenomenon. Ignorance won't do.

CHAPTER 8

The 'mouldy' patient

Undoubtedly one of the biggest breakthroughs in the field of allergy and ecological medicine has been the recognition of the role played by the organism CANDIDA ALBICANS. First reported in 1978 by Orian Truss, an American holistic psychiatrist, it has risen steadily in importance in clinical ecology practice until now I find it is relevant to over a third of my patients. Some of my colleagues would put its incidence far higher than this. However, there is, to date, no creditable scientific test for the problem described in this chapter and so the exact frequency must remain merely speculation.

The important point is that Candida albicans is only part of the whole picture. Just as it may not be possible for a patient with allergies to get well without eradicating Candida, it is also not possible to recover fully merely treating Candida, without also cleaning up the patient's environment, eliminating food allergies and correcting nutritional imbalances. It is important to see the overall view and realize that Candida is basically an effect and not a cause as some enthusiastic writers might suggest.

What is it?

Candida albicans is a yeast-like germ that causes Thrush. However we are not talking here about the infection which occurs so commonly in babies' mouths and women's vaginas but a rather more serious colonization deep within the bowel. From there, it works its mischief indirectly and seems able actually to generate food and chemical intolerances, probably by increasing the total body load and perhaps even suppressing the immune system.

It is a problem very much of our modern age, largely caused by doctors themselves, as you will see. In fact you may feel that it is a considerable price to pay for the supposed wonders of drug therapy. The result is that we now have almost a Candida epidemic and we may be damaging our internal environment in much the same crazy way we are looting the earth, eroding soil and destroying rain forests to alter, irreversibly, the relationship of Man with the environment on which he depends so much.

When is a yeast not a yeast?

As already pointed out, Candida albicans is in the yeast family of organisms. That means it ferments sugars to make alcohol and lives on the energy released in this process.

In fact there are cases on record of people actually drunk from large amounts of alcohol produced in this way — that is, without having imbibed any alcoholic drink. This is sufficiently well recognized that courts of law have, in a few rare cases, accepted it as a valid defence against a charge of drinking and driving (the individuals concerned were able to prove beyond reasonable doubt that they had not been drinking but that they *did* have Candida albicans).

It exists in more than one form and in the bowel it takes on a vegetative phase, from which grow thread-like extensions (hyphae). These are able to penetrate the cell lining of the gut and from there it becomes very difficult to dislodge.

Somehow, it seems to generate or enhance food intolerance. One mechanism which has been suggested is that it allows toxins from the bowel to escape through the gut wall into the bloodstream. The contents of the bowel are particularly likely to make an individual unwell, as anyone who suffers from constipation can testify.

Even more strikingly, Candida seems to have the power to cause heightened chemical sensitivity and, so far, this is impossible to explain.

Predisposing factors

Almost all human Candida infections come from other human beings. However, the mere presence of the organism does not automatically lead to the overgrowth of Candida within the bowel.

Certain predisposing factors to favour this occurrence must be present for it to take place.

Briefly speaking, anything which suppresses natural immunity will increase the likelihood of Candida becoming established. I mentioned the abuse of medical drugs. Three groups of medicines are outstanding in this respect:

- corticosteroids

- the Pill and other oestrogen hormones

- broad-spectrum antibiotics

The latter are by far the commonest. Few children in the last two or three decades have not been dosed repeatedly for colds and sore throats with penicillin or its many equivalents. Often the general practitioner prescribes the broad-spectrum type as a sort of catch-all. This is ignorance and folly of the highest order.

To begin with, most of these upper respiratory tract infections are caused by viruses, which are quite unharmed by any antibiotic. Secondly, the wide-acting antibiotics kill off normal safe friendly germs which live in our bowel and on which we depend for health. The presence of these 'natural germs' is a kind of in-built immunity against infections by their more unpleasant 'wild' counterparts, which cause disease. Once these are killed or harmed, the way is clear for Candida and other pathogenic (disease-causing) organisms to take over. This may be of little consequence if the antibiotic saves your life, but in common everyday situations, where the use of an antibiotic is not really called for, the price may be too high.

Steroid drugs work by suppressing the body's immune defence mechanisms. This can have benefit in certain diseases, such as asthma, which are caused by allergy. But in the process, loss of immunity allows attack by many diseases, of which Candida is only one. Remember AIDS is nothing more than a loss of the body's immunity and fatal overwhelming infections, Candida included, are the inevitable result. One would logically tamper with this process therefore only with extreme caution.

On a similar topic, certain natural disease processes, other than acquired immune deficiency syndrome, also retard immunity, and in this respect leukaemias and related cancers have long been known. These conditions are beyond the scope of this simple book.

More recent is the emergence, or rather the recognition, of myalgic encephalomyelitis (see Chapter 9).

Finally, there is evidence to suggest that the birth-control pill predisposes to Candida. This might be due in part to increased sexual activity in women on the Pill but it is often forgotten that sex hormones are also steroid substances. It could be more than a coincidence that since the introduction of the Pill and its very widespread use by Western women, there has been an alarming increase in the incidence of Candida.

I'm referring now to intestinal Candida, not the obvious vaginal infections. In fact these may be a secondary phenomenon, the woman constantly re-infecting herself from her own nearby anus.

Diet

It is impossible not to suspect that another major contributory cause to Candida infection is our bad modern diet, with its great excess of refined carbohydrates, sugars in particular.

Coincident with the rise in the use of antibiotics and modern drugs has been the switch to supermarket 'junk' or prepackaged foods. While there is no direct evidence that this can lead to Candida it is unlikely that food manufacturing companies will provide the money and research facilities needed to investigate this sort of problem. So, for the moment at least, it must remain no more than a hypothesis.

But in the meantime, if you'll settle for an informed opinion (no more), it is very probable that diet plays an important part in the origination of Candida overgrowth. (See Box 23.)

Diagnosis

Candida is a great mimic. It causes a myriad of symptoms, directly and also indirectly, through provoking complex multiple food and chemical intolerances. Many of these symptoms are hard to define; some are extremely bizarre; some are highly subjective and likely to lead to the patient being accused of being neurotic or 'imaginative'.

However, certain special symptoms seem to point very strongly to the presence of Candida in the gut. Three I used to call the Terrible Trio:

BOX 23

The bio-ecology of Candida albicans

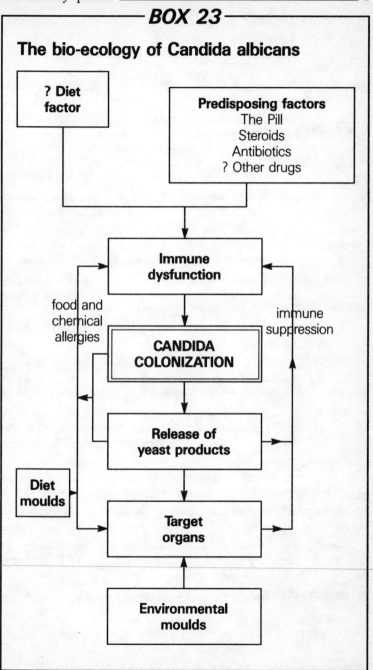

- craving for sweet things
- alcohol intolerance
- chemical sensitivity

To these I have now added:

- bloating

Perhaps I should call this the Awesome Foursome! Two out of four from this list means Candida is highly probable. With three or all of them it makes it a virtual certainty.

Two other very important symptoms caused by Candida, though not diagnostic, are excessive fatigue and depression (a sort of grinding apathy).

Supporting symptoms include mould sensitivity (patient worse on damp days, in musty, damp or old surroundings) and the presence of known fungal infection, either in the skin (such as athlete's foot) or Candida itself, in the mouth or vagina.

Lastly, one or more of the predisposing factors referred to above is usually present in the patient's history.

What is lacking is a credible scientific test for the presence of Candida. It has been suggested that we could starve the patient of carbohydrates for a few days, measure the patient's blood alcohol level, then give a test feed of sugars. A repeat of the blood alcohol test a few hours later, if raised, would show the presence of fermenting organisms within the bowel. Perhaps this test will become established one day.

In the meantime, we have to rely on what is known as a therapeutic trial. That is, the patient is put on the appropriate treatment. If it works, he or she is then presumed to have had the disease. This isn't quite as crude as it sounds. Much modern so-called scientific medicine is done this way. After many tests, X-rays etc., when nothing concrete is found, it is common practice to prescribe a drug speculatively, to see if it works.

The therapeutic trial leads naturally on to the subject of treatment.

Treatment

Optimum therapy for Candida has four main aspects:

- Nystatin and other drugs

- avoidance of sugar and refined carbohydrate

- avoiding mould (yeast) foods

- Lactobacillus acidophilus supplements

Only one of these, the prescription-only medicine NYSTATIN or similar, cannot be carried out by the individual concerned. The other three are simple dietary remedies. Thus if you suspect you have Candida, even if your own doctor will not co-operate, you can at least reduce it and keep it in check, without too much difficulty.

Nystatin and other drugs

Nystatin is a yellow-green, foul-tasting powder. Generally the dose will be set by the physician but the wise practitioner will allow the patient a certain amount of leeway to adjust the dose for optimum effect. Too little seems to result in increased lethargy, too much can cause jumpiness and irritability.

Initially the dose is 4,000,000–8,000,000IU daily (1,000,000IU is equal to a quarter of a teaspoon).

It is important to note that, although Nystatin has long been available in tablet and pessary form, these are little help in this situation. Tablets don't break up until reaching the stomach and so leave the mouth largely untreated. This remains a reservoir of Candida, which continues to re-infect the lower gut from above, so the condition never properly clears.

Fortunately, though most surprisingly, allergy patients seem to tolerate Nystatin quite well. Perhaps this is because it is so insoluble; hardly any finds its way into the blood-stream. There may be disagreeable side-effects at first, but after that it usually causes no difficulty. This early reaction we think may be due to killing off Candida in large numbers. The debris will be digested and toxins released. It's a plausible theory, though merely speculative.

Those who can't tolerate Nystatin should experiment with a varied dose before abandoning it entirely. Sometimes taking smaller amounts, or dosing only on certain days of the week will enable it to be included in the programme in a limited way. This is truly a case where 'every little helps'.

There are alternative drugs to Nystatin but these are not so safe.

Amphotericin is probably the least risky. Ketoconazole may also be used, at the discretion of the physician. I never prescribe it.

Candida is an extremely tenacious organism and it may be necessary to continue taking the Nystatin for many months. I always take the patient off it after a maximum of six months. I believe it is an important principle to let Nature try to regain control.

Avoid sugar

To avoid fermenting organisms such as yeasts it is necessary to deny them sugar. This means cakes, biscuits, sweets, chocolate bars, etc. In my opinion, it is *not* important to avoid natural foods containing sugar, such as fruit, though I do limit dried fruit (which is not natural, of course).

To do otherwise is to feed the Candida and this is illogical, to say the least. Not that a small amount of sugar need be avoided like poison — a sprinkle on cooking apples or rhubarb, for instance, won't do any real harm. It's a quantitative thing. This is emphasized because there are one or two very extreme 'Candida' diets being pressed upon the public, principally by non-doctors, who do not properly understand nutrition.

Avoid yeast-like foods

It is also important to avoid yeast-like or 'mould' foods. Such foods include:

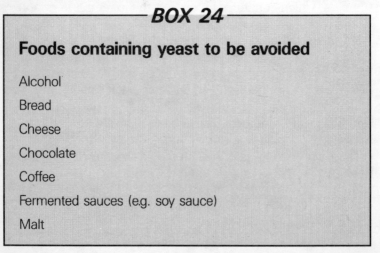

BOX 24

Foods containing yeast to be avoided

Alcohol

Bread

Cheese

Chocolate

Coffee

Fermented sauces (e.g. soy sauce)

Malt

BOX 24

Foods containing yeast to be avoided (cont)

Mushrooms and other fungi

Vinegar

Vitamin B from natural sources

Note: Fruit juices, unless freshly squeezed, can contain significant amounts of natural yeast. Over-ripe and obviously mouldy food is, of course, unsuitable.

A number of other specialized foods, such as pretzels, may also contain yeast.

All of these foods are likely to make the patient with Candida feel generally unwell. Also, he or she will notice that musty old buildings and damp days (with a high incidence of mould in the air) cause symptoms to recur. Hence the jocular expression 'mouldy' patient.

Re-colonizing the bowel

If you fully understand the introductory paragraphs of this chapter, you will readily see it makes sense to try and repopulate the bowel with harmless, 'friendly' germs.

Chief among these are the yogurt bacteria LACTOBACILLUS ACIDOPHILUS and L. BULGARICUS, which are now readily available as diet supplements. The purer brands tend to be expensive. Those products which appear cheaper are often simply diluted with lactose (milk sugar) which may be very unsuitable for those with lactose intolerance.

Strictly dairy-free brands are available but not easy to obtain.

Capricin

Capricin is the registered brand name of an entirely new approach to Candida control, marketed by Professional Services Inc. of California, USA.

Certain naturally occurring substances inhibit the growth of Candida. One of these is malic acid, found in the vagina. Candida *never* becomes tolerant or resistant to this substance and it is Nature's own way of preventing permanent serious thrush vaginitis (instances of vaginal thrush are all attributable to an upset in the natural fluids, causing the acidity to be temporarily lost).

A similar long-chain acid occurs in the bowel, called caprilic acid. It too inhibits the growth of Candida and other unwanted pathogens in the bowel but not bacteria like Lactobacillus, which thrives happily in acid surroundings.

In its natural state, caprilic acid is rather noxious. Now a clever biochemist has succeeded in taming it and rendering it harmless but not ineffective, in capsule form. It can be bought as a dietary supplement, that is without prescription. Other brands will probably follow.

It is fairly well tolerated, can be taken for long periods and also may be used in conjunction with Nystatin, or on its own.

Vaginal thrush

Vaginal thrush is altogether a different problem, though not unnaturally the two may exist side by side.

In treating intestinal Candidiasis with Nystatin, this has little or no effect on the vaginal infection. Indeed, it may sometimes make it worse, an observation I have made many times but without any satisfactory explanation as to why.

Instead, this condition needs its own specific treatment, using Nystatin pessaries. It is prudent also to treat the woman's sexual partner with a cream. Otherwise he will simply keep reinfecting her.

The probable reason oral Nystatin doesn't help the vaginal condition is that the substance in its powder form is almost insoluble. It does not get into the bloodstream and does not get carried around the body in the way that, say, an antibiotic does.

Of course, properly treated intestinal Candida will remove a potential source of re-infection of the vagina. If the male partner is treated at the same time, this should go a long way to preventing re-infection, once clear.

Attention to these important points in prescribing is not common among practitioners and consequently a lot of women suffer needlessly.

Recurrence

Once treated, what is to stop a patient getting intestinal thrush all over again?

Nothing at all.

In fact it is bound to happen, unless attention is given to the bio-ecology of yeasts, as discussed in this chapter. Thus, if the patient needs to be given a course of broad-spectrum antibiotics, Candida is likely to be triggered once more. Once the immune system has been weakened, as in an allergic patient, infection is a constant hazard.

However, it can be said that in the overwhelming majority of people who suffer this complaint, care with the diet, an intelligent use of bowel flora supplementation and vitamins to strengthen the immune system (as described in Chapter 6) prevent any further trouble.

The trick is to let Nature resume control and get everything balanced properly once more. For this reason, I condemn the continued use of Nystatin and other antifungals; longer than about six months simply shouldn't be necessary. Frequent recurrence usually means that some other aspect of the management of Candida is being neglected.

If some crisis directs the use of antibiotics — and in some situations this may be vital — Nystatin can always be taken concurrently or subsequently, to prevent the re-establishment of Candida.

CHAPTER 9

Post-viral fatigue syndrome

It is appropriate to bring in a discussion of this condition even in a modest volume of this size. To begin with, I think it is very common indeed and simply not being diagnosed and secondly, it is very relevant to the study of allergy — indeed ultimate comprehension of post-viral fatigue syndrome will, I am convinced, enrich our understanding of allergy. We may learn what the real mechanism is, how it comes about and how best to treat it. Lastly, in a world poised anxiously perhaps on the brink of a catastrophic AIDS epidemic there are similarities in both diseases and perhaps lessons to be learned.

What's in a name?

The condition has a number of names including Royal Free Disease, Tapanui 'Flu and Iceland Disease, commemorating what seem to have been epidemic outbreaks in various parts of the world. Myalgic encephalomyelitis is the official term in the UK, meaning muscle pain and brain inflammation, which is a good description of the condition. In the USA epidemic neuromyasthenia is the term preferred by doctors, while the American public know it as chronic Epstein-Barr virus (CEBV); but this is rather premature since the causative agent has not been properly identified and among UK doctors it is thought not likely to be the Epstein-Barr virus. I prefer post-viral fatigue syndrome (PVFS) since it isn't so pretentious and its significance can be understood by the layman.

The disadvantage in this term is that a great many people seem to have the disease *without* being able to relate it to an acute viral attack. Possibly their illness began with a mild unobserved viral episode. Perhaps we are wide of the mark on what the origin of this condition really is and a viral episode may only be the first identifiable aspect of the illness, not the cause at all.

PVFS is a clinical syndrome; that is, a collection of symptoms, rather than a disease entity, so even its very existence is hotly debated by members of the medical profession. Many doctors prefer to think in psychiatric terms; indeed, even outbreaks of epidemic proportions do not deter them from this view which they deem to be 'mass hysteria'.

The search is currently on to identify a guilty virus. In some ways I am apprehensive about this because there may well be a number of viruses to blame and the danger is that when one is identified, others will be ignored and patients who don't have the 'official' version will be dismissed as neurotic.

Clinical presentation

The disease seems to have all the hallmarks of a chronic viral illness. Very little is known about the acute phase because, except in the

---

BOX 25

Some symptoms at onset of PVFS

Abdominal pain

Dizziness

Double vision

Headache

Lassitude, inertia

Low grade fever (can be absent)

Muscle weakness

Nausea or vomiting

Pains in neck, back or limbs

Pins and needles

Sore throat

Tinnitus

case of an epidemic, it isn't usually recognized for what it is. By the time the disease is identified, it has moved into the chronic phase. All we do know is that the central nervous system is significantly affected and the frequency of associated sore throat and upper respiratory tract infection suggests the probable port of entry is through inhalation of infected moisture droplets (Box 25).

The chronic stage can give rise to a vast array of symptoms, very much like a long-term allergy, with many target organs. However certain symptoms seem to be outstanding in frequency and severity. Most important is FATIGUE (hence the name). It is no ordinary fatigue but has a very characteristic pattern. The victim functions normally up to a certain threshold. Any exertion beyond this level has severe consequences; thus, for example, playing one set of tennis may be perfectly fine, but two sets would put the victim in bed for a day or two. The unfortunate consequence of this is that the victim appears normal in most situations but because of limitations has to curtail activity drastically. To other people this seems no more than laziness in a person who is perfectly healthy and given to hypochondria.

The second most important symptom is DEPRESSION: heavy black gloom which comes in fits and starts. There may be frightening nightmares. Usually the dread and anxiety is altogether

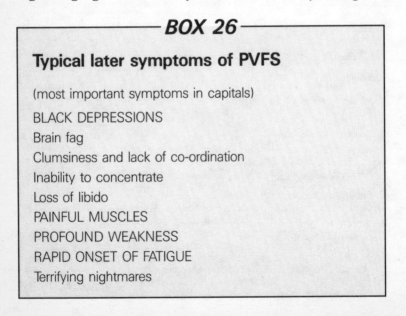

BOX 26

Typical later symptoms of PVFS

(most important symptoms in capitals)

BLACK DEPRESSIONS

Brain fag

Clumsiness and lack of co-ordination

Inability to concentrate

Loss of libido

PAINFUL MUSCLES

PROFOUND WEAKNESS

RAPID ONSET OF FATIGUE

Terrifying nightmares

inappropriate and friends and relatives are frequently upset to find a formerly cheerful individual become morose, withdrawn and apathetic for no apparent reason. This puts immense strain on inter-personal relations which is bound to make matters worse.

A number of other symptoms occur with regular frequency. Probably almost any altered perception is possible, due to cerebral irritation (Box 26).

Which virus?

The two most likely culprits known are the Epstein-Barr virus, well known for its potential for lingering illness (glandular fever) and Coxsackie B which, technically speaking, is a most unlikely candidate for this sort of illness, yet it seems to turn up suspiciously often.

Recently, enteroviruses of the polio type have been implicated. This makes particular sense as these viruses are known to attack the nervous system. Some of the microscopic spinal cord changes in PVFS are similar to early stages of polio. Tests are continuing.

As you will see in the next section, even the commonplace influenza virus could not be excluded from suspicion; in the right circumstances, it can be an extremely destructive pathogen of Man.

Possibly an as-yet unidentified virus is to blame. This is perfectly feasible as new strains arrive from time to time, as with the AIDS virus, for example. The important point to make is that a great many sufferers with this condition can give no firm history of a viral type illness at the onset of their condition — probably the majority cannot.

Search for a model

PVFS is a poorly understood condition, if it exists at all. Even so, it is never too early to search for a model which might explain what is happening to sufferers and, possibly, give us insight into how to deal with it. Such objective serological findings as there may be seem to point to a chronic virus attack which the body is somehow unable to shrug off. It is as if the infection attacks and impairs the immune system itself and so handicaps the ability to fight back. Here there is a strong similarity with AIDS.

Reading the work of Professor Linus Businco in Italy, it struck me that he had uncovered a very workable model of PVFS. He took a population of guinea pigs and subjected them to daily inhalations of a mixture of Hong Kong, Texas and USSR strains of influenza virus. He slaughtered samples at 10, 20 and 30 days and compared the findings on these animals with controls which had not received the virus doses.

The results were quite startling, to say the least. He found massive widespread damage to the internal organs. There was atrophy and fibrosis of the heart, lungs, liver, thyroid, lymph tissue and testes. Worse: the adrenal glands had actually haemorrhaged on many specimens, so bad was the damage. It is impossible to imagine that a body attacked in this way does not suffer a considerable loss of function, especially loss of immune potential. Remember these were 'everyday' viruses, not hitherto known for organ destruction capability. The difference in this experiment was simply that the animals were not permitted to shrug off the virus attack, but subjected to it daily for a matter of some weeks. Could this happen to human beings also unable to rid themselves of pathogenic viruses?

Professor Businco's findings are fascinating and very disconcerting indeed.

Diagnosis

One of the problems that has plagued investigation into PVFS and a major reason it remains in dispute is that there is no satisfactory test to say whether or not a patient is suffering from it. Until the time comes when there is such a test, nobody knows for sure what alters and thus what to measure.

Dr Patrick Behan in Glasgow set out to find what changes, if any, could be detected in a typical group of PVFS cases from a local outbreak among doctors, students and nurses. He and his team screened 50 cases, carrying out tests on the blood, muscles, nervous tissue and immune system and comparing the results with the same tests carried out on 50 controls, most of whom were healthy but also included were certain similar conditions, such as motor neurone disease, myasthenia gravis, meningitis and alcoholic nerve damage.

Among the positive findings was a clear-cut proof of actual muscle weakness. It followed the exact pattern described earlier, that is, it only came after exertion and was then profound. In some cases, quite marked incapacity resulted from even mild effort, such as climbing 40 stairs. This was further backed up by electromyographic changes, that is, disorder in the way that nerve transmission is passed to the muscles.

There was increased blood viscosity ('stickiness'), which could account for loss of brain function.

Most striking of all was change in the circulating lymphocytes. This was highly abnormal in 35 of the 50 cases. The best way of summarizing this is by means of a table (Box 27). The T-helper cells, those which have positive immune benefit, are considerably reduced and T-suppressor cells, *those which reduce immunity*, were allowed to work unchecked. Row 1 shows the acute stage of the illness, row 2 the pattern of chronic ME. For your interest I have added available information on AIDS (row 3), which you can see is strikingly similar to ME. Natural killer cells (highly beneficial germ-killers) are unchanged in ME whereas these are lost in AIDS, with serious consequences.

BOX 27

Lymphocyte changes in chronic ME (PVFS) compared with AIDS

	Total lymphocytes	Suppressor lymphocytes	Helper lymphocytes	Ratio	Natural killer cells
1 Acute ME	↓	↓	Normal	↓	Normal
2 Chronic ME	↓	Normal	↓	↓	Normal
3 AIDS	↓	Normal	↓	↓	↓

(↓) means lowered.

Apart from Dr Behan's work, the other main changes which have been associated with PVFS are raised serum complement C1, which is simply a sign of ongoing virus infection and isn't specific to this condition and the often-reported increase in anti-Coxsackie B antibodies.

The ME Association reports that 85 per cent of cases have important anti-Coxsackie B levels. Other workers say there isn't any difference between ME cases and the normal population, many of whom have had a Coxsackie infection and recovered entirely.

Intensive research is presently going on and no doubt the picture will clarify in time.

Treatment

The 'official' view, that is the opinion of those who think they are experts in this condition, is that it slowly gets better. This may be true of a small percentage of cases, but for the majority, the prognosis is fairly bleak. The disease does not improve and may, in fact, slowly get worse. Once the disease becomes established, and in the absence of any intervention, it is probably permanent.

However, that does not mean that it isn't treatable. What strikes the modern allergist about this condition is how like the allergy syndrome it manifests. Whatever the cause of PVFS and the underlying mechanism of its effect, the final result is that the victim suffers with multiple food and chemical intolerances. This is the key that opens the door to successful treatment.

It would be appropriate, therefore, for an ME sufferer to begin with a routine exclusion diet and challenge tests. I do not recommend fasting; this can cause serious difficulties. A rotation diet of varied safe foods is the best long-term protection against food allergies.

Very few sufferers would not benefit from a chemical clean-up of the home and work environment, as described in Chapter 5. Anything which reduces the body load in this way is bound to help. Thus rest, recreation and fresh-air are 'valid' treatments.

Vitamins and minerals seem to help greatly. Guidelines are given in Chapter 6 for strengthening the immune system in this way.

Candida is a very common concomitant of PVFS. This is not surprising, since the immune system is impaired. We call this an opportunistic infection and here again there is a strong similarity with AIDS, though in PVFS these never reach the same life-threatening proportions. Treatment would proceed exactly as in Chapter 8.

Some progress with treatment can be made on a self-help basis, though it must be admitted results are much more certain if professional advice is sought from someone who understands what to do. I find Miller's provocation and neutralizing method of enormous help in sifting through the complex sensitivities and treating them. Chemical allergy can be the worst aspect of this condition and usually neutralizing drops are necessary to cope with our increasingly hostile environment.

Drug treatment of PVFS is a failure. Attempts to use gamma-globulin injection are similarly worthless overall.

Long-term prospects

It is very important that PVFS victims keep a positive attitude. It is all too easy to retreat into a shell, avoid human company and fade away indoors. Once this psychological deficit becomes established, it is very hard to break, even with expert help from a doctor with the skill to alleviate the worst of the symptoms and it will, of course, limit recovery. This gives rise to the conviction, among outsiders, that the patient doesn't actually want to get well.

Recovery is generally very slow and much patience is needed. Early improvement, on the proper programme, should be quite normal but it may take up to six months to get maximum benefit, perhaps longer. Also, it must be said that total recovery is very rare. Probably the least responsive symptom is that characteristic fatigue. I have many PVFS patients who feel well and now lead happy, productive lives but their exercise tolerance has not returned. Some do better than others, but in general improvement in this respect is only slight.

In the meantime, psychological support from family and friends is very important. By my experience, the single most valued help for sufferers is just that somebody believes they are ill. For many, the burden of their affliction is made intolerably worse by the fact that nobody acknowledges the illness for what it is and the victims are written off as idle, morbid, egocentric, neurotic, or all of these. Doctors are often quick to offend in this way.

Yet, while in the grip of a frightening — almost nightmare — illness, scorn is the last thing you need.

CHAPTER 10

The mercury hazard: fact or fiction?

Much concern has been expressed in recent years about the dangers of mercury from dental fillings. It is true to say that a lot of wild opinion is being heralded as fact and so much is being claimed by champions of this newly recognized hazard, that their over-enthusiasm is tending to create disbelief. This is a pity, because if it is indeed a danger to health, then the sooner it is widely recognized the better. Extremism is definitely counter-productive.

This chapter attempts to be an objective overview of the evidence, from which the reader must make up his or her own mind where the truth lies. I have tried to distinguish between fact and theory, though it must be understood that what today is supposition may tomorrow be scientific fact.

The biochemistry of mercury

It is indisputable that mercury is a heavy metal, liquid at ordinary temperatures, but which vaporizes easily and can be inhaled. It is absorbed readily by human tissues and seems to have a special affinity for the nervous system and brain, which it damages rather easily.

Mild symptoms may include forgetfulness, confusion and disorientation. More serious prolonged exposure can bring on tremor and permanent mental changes. The most extreme form of mercury poisoning leads to psychosis and wild jerking spasms of the limbs. In the old days this was seen frequently in workers making hat-bands, which were cured with mercuric chloride: hence the expression, 'Mad as a hatter'. In more modern times it has recurred as Minamata disease, named after a town in Japan, where many of the population were poisoned by mercury effluvia from a factory, which contaminated fish in the local bay. These degenerations are, unfortunately, irreversible.

Some individuals have an allergic hypersensitivity to mercury, and various estimates place this between 1 and 15 per cent of the population. It seems to increase with exposure. Testing with patch tests (see below) is much more likely to be positive after five years of exposure. It is interesting to report that dental students, working with mercury amalgam, show a sharp increase in reaction to it as they progress through their studies.

In passing, it should be noted that similar sensitivities can occur with other metals, notably nickel, chromium, cobalt and gold. Apart from nickel, these are exceptionally rare. Nevertheless, they are not excluded from remarks made in this chapter.

Mercury in dental fillings

For over 100 years mercury in dental fillings (amalgam) was felt to be completely safe. After all, the metal is cast in a solid form, which stays *in situ* in the tooth, out of harm's way. Doesn't it?

Well, not quite. In certain circumstances it is slowly leached out of the tooth. The amounts may only be very small but we are talking now about allergy: very tiny amounts can wreak havoc. The surprise reason for the release of the metal in its natural state, entirely unthought of until the last few years, is electrolysis, that is the electrical dissolving of metal. Amalgam-filled teeth can actually act as tiny batteries and give off a current. This can be measured with a potentiometer by simply placing one electrode over the affected filling. Exposure of the inside of such teeth shows oxidation (scorch) marks where the current has flowed over many years. There may be gaps where the amalgam has simply dissolved away.

So, far from being safe, having dental fillings is rather like sucking a mercury lozenge continuously. We know that mercury is very poisonous. So perhaps it shouldn't be surprising, after all, that it may be making some of us sick.

The symptoms

The symptoms due to mercury allergy (as opposed to toxicity, which is described above) can be many and varied. In fact the range of effects covers all target organs, from skin rashes and bowel disturbance, to asthma and mood changes. It seems to contribute to the allergy problem, probably by adding to the body load, so any allergy symptom can be prolonged or made worse by it. Suppression of the immune system (see below) ties it in to Candida overgrowth and it may be difficult to eradicate this organism without attending to the possibility of mercury poisoning.

It is important to think of mercury in any allergy case not responding to proper treatment. This is especially important in degenerative and auto-immune diseases, such as multiple sclerosis, lupus erythematosis, rheumatoid arthritis, colitis and arteriosclerosis (hardening of the arteries). Also any vague mental symptoms, not responding to other treatment, such as lethargy, depression, loss of memory, etc. might well begin to recover after removal of toxic mercury.

Tests

We are devilled by the lack of a good objective test to show whether or not the patient is reacting to mercury.

The only standardized 'scientific' test for mercury allergy is patch testing. However, it is very unreliable and, although positive results may be helpful, negative ones do not exclude the presence of significant reactions. In any case, it may be possible to demonstrate a sensitivity to mercury but that still doesn't tell us whether it is directly making the person sick or not.

A blood profile, though not specific to mercury poisoning, may help. If the general level of lymphocytes is low or the ratio of helper to suppressor lymphocytes is far from what it should be, this is evidence of immune suppression (AIDS and myalgic encephalomyelitis also produce this change). *In the absence of any other reason* for a decline in lymphocyte population, it is vital to consider mercury poisoning as a possible cause.

Loss of functioning lymphocytes is one of the reasons an individual may experience food and other allergies. Not surprisingly, if mercury fillings are removed and the lymphocytes correct themselves (as usually happens), then the allergies will also improve. Thus, some patients, after having their fillings changed, find themselves able to eat certain foods that for years they could not.

This doesn't *prove* anything, but it fits with the hypothesis and is therefore supportive of it.

Other tests have been suggested, but few of these would be accepted, even by unconventional doctors. It remains to be seen whether faith in them is justified. The Vega machine may give a positive reading but since mercury is a known poison, it could be argued that this advances the case very little. Applied kinesiology may also show a provoked muscle weakness, when the patient is tested with mercury.

I have also been told, in good faith, that the latter test may be carried out by having the patient make direct contact with the dental fillings and that will also react positively, if mercury is a problem to that patient. As elsewhere in this chapter, you are asked to make up your own mind as to the validity or otherwise of these tests. However, it must be borne in mind that the positive reactions on these tests can be reproduced over and over, even done 'blind': that is, without the doctor or patient knowing what is in the test phial, the mercury shows up each time.

Homoeopathy

Jack Levenson, a holistic dentist, has suggested a different sort of test for which he claims good results, though he isn't rash enough to suggest it is more than a guide. If the patient is given a test dose of homoeopathic Merc. Sol. 30, it may produce a temporary improvement. This is a good indication that the patient will benefit from having mercury amalgams removed. A single dose of vitamin B_1, if it lifts fatigue dramatically, may have the same implication.

One of the problems is assessing what is meant by improvement. It is well known that patients may get a false sense of benefit during a test, the so-called placebo effect. To avoid this, the test should be done double-blind, that is with several tablets, only one of which is the real test substance. The tablets are coded and only *after* the results have been reported is the code broken and the test assessment made.

I have tried this using what is called a 10cm line test to grade the responses. Briefly, when the symptom being reported is somewhat vague (how can you grade 'Feeling I can't go on', for example?), the 10cm line test is accepted by scientific workers as a valid means of putting a numerical value to the result.

The patient is asked to consider a line 10cm (4 inches) long as representing all grades of symptoms from absent on the left side to as severe as imaginable on the right. He or she then makes a mark along this scale which represents how he or she feels at that precise moment. Towards the right would suggest quite unpleasant feelings, towards the left would mean feeling reasonably well. It is then a simple matter to measure the relative proportions along this line as a numerical value of 'feeling'. This can be done for one symptom only, or several simultaneously (a different graph for each).

It works far better than asking the patient, 'On a scale of 1 to 10, how do you feel?' This sort of question can be difficult to answer and the finer shades of sensation, half scores, etc. can intimidate the patient and prevent an accurate score. The 10cm line test seems

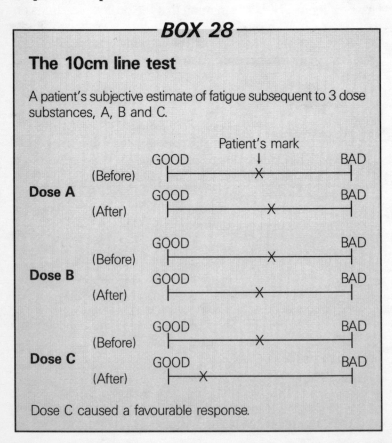

BOX 28

The 10cm line test

A patient's subjective estimate of fatigue subsequent to 3 dose substances, A, B and C.

Dose C caused a favourable response.

to get round these difficulties very neatly.

So for the mercury test, the patient takes a number of tablets, at intervals of several days, scoring the line test before and after each. If the one which shows improvement is the active substance and not a 'blank', the test is considered positive (see Box 28).

Treatment

If it is decided with confidence that mercury is indeed a problem, the solution is relatively straightforward — remove the mercury. I say 'relatively' because removing dental amalgams and replacing them with porcelain or other composite substitutes is not altogether easy. To begin with, it is not available now, or in the foreseeable future, on the National Health Service and is an expensive treatment, the cost of which must be borne entirely by the patient.

Also the substitute fillings can be a source of great difficulties if not put in with considerable care. It takes a special skill which probably not every dentist has, even if he were willing to undertake such a course of treatment.

During the operation, the dentist must use a rubber dam around the tooth while he works on it, in order to prevent spillage of mercury into the patient's mouth as the removal progresses.

Finally, it is possible, with the greatest technical ability available, to make a patient worse while removing the mercury fillings. Experts say this will happen often *unless the fillings are replaced in the correct sequence.*

The key to this is the electrical readings which are obtained from the distressed amalgam. It is important to start with the tooth giving the strongest negative electrical potential, then take the next, then the next and so on. To do otherwise could have serious consequences.

Even when successful, recovery may still take many months after the conclusion of treatment.

General mercury load

As well as the considerable quantity of mercury found in fillings, the body may carry amounts within the tissues. This is (hopefully) less in quantity but more serious for health. Probably the main source of this tissue mercury is dental work but another important source is fungicides containing mercury, which happens through consuming crops treated by this means, and eating contaminated fish. There are less common sources, which need not concern us here.

It is wise to try to reduce this body burden of mercury. Jack Levenson recommends homoeopathic Merc. Sol. 30 or Hepar Sulph. 30. Taking anti-oxidising vitamins (A, E and C) helps, also selenium. Kelp may be used, which contains sodium alginate, a chelating compound which draws mercury (and other heavy metals, such as lead) from the system. Also zinc will tend to displace such heavy metals reasonably safely.

Special injections (EDTA), under strict medical control, may be necessary if the mercury poisoning comes from a large dose, such as occupational exposure. All the above supplements would remain valid in this situation.

EDTA provocation test

If the case is serious enough to warrant it (EDTA is rather risky and should not be used lightly), EDTA can be used to test the patient for mercury within the body. A preliminary 24-hour urine sample is taken and its mercury content (if any) measured. The EDTA dose is then administered and a further 24-hour urine sample collected. If mercury appears in the urine after the challenge, it implies it exists widely within the body.

The type of patients to consider for this test are those with poor lymphocyte counts or with unresponding auto-immune disease, not improving after the removal of mercury amalgams.

Naturally, if the test proves positive, the patient should be given a series of such injections, until no more mercury can be detected in the urine samples. At this time, it is presumed the body is reasonably clear. More accurately, whatever mercury remains in the body is chemically bound up and can't be removed.

Conclusion

That's about all there is to our knowledge about mercury and allergies. Not much, I think you'll agree. The evidence is scanty, but doctors working in this field have a steadily increasing casebook of successful recoveries, cases which were simply not getting better any other way, *until the mercury problem was addressed*. Why wait for scientific 'proof' if you might be one of these lucky cases?

The choice really rests with the patient. Given the facts and the doubts presented here, he or she must simply decide where the truth lies. Generally speaking, little harm can come from removing mercury fillings *providing it is done properly* and the results could be well worthwhile. If you accept that it is expensive and might not work but would like to try, go ahead. That's the only sensible advice to give.

CHAPTER 11

Light as food

Most of us are happier, more cheerful and energetic during the summer months. The long, lazy, sunny days seem to bring out the best in us. Winter is a time of greater ill-health, moody introversion and a tendency to withdraw from life.

Instinctively, we associate this with animal hibernation. In the higher latitudes of the northern hemisphere, the climate is too severe for much activity and animal life tends to reduce to the merest essentials, food and sleep. There are long periods of inactivity. In its most extreme form, winter is passed in a deep metabolic coma, awakened only by the returning warmth of spring.

Human beings, of course, don't hibernate in this way. We're far too advanced. Besides, we have fire.

Well, it seems that we are not quite free of the natural biological cycle. Remarkable studies in recent years have shown that diminution in the surrounding light levels can result in a drop-off in mental activity. This might be hardly noticeable for most of us. But for some people it can mean significant depression. Because it is thought to be seasonal and the medical word for mood is affect, this postulated condition is called seasonal affective disorder, or SAD for short.

Since it is an environmental condition, it is discussed in brief here.

Research

Links between health and light have been understood for a long time. For example, sunlight on the skin is known to be one of the sources of vitamin D. Rickets became very common in large cities, where smoky atmosphere cut off the sun, before the vitamin D connection was discovered and smoke-free regulations helped to solve the problem. Light also helps clear jaundice in the newborn child. Fluorescent lighting gives many people headaches, blurred vision and can be responsible for depleting vitamin A within the body.

However, the realization that light is important to mood has been slow in coming. Now psychiatrists in the USA and Britain have carried out studies that seem to prove the existence of SAD. Adults suffer primarily from depression, lethargy and overeating. Children, it appears, tend more towards lack of sleep, irritability and withdrawal. The effect on school performance can be quite detrimental.

It is important, in considering 'winter depression', to rule out other factors, such as the gradual loss of key vitamins from foodstuffs as the sun declines. However, even allowing for such factors, it seems that we are on the edge of a new breakthrough in our understanding of ourselves and the healthy functioning of our bodies.

We are nowadays used to the idea of 'biological clocks'. The menstrual cycle of women clearly originated from phases of the moon. It seems quite logical therefore that the sun, so much more powerful and dominating, should also have regulating effects. In fact researches implicate solar radiation levels in controlling, or at least influencing, endocrine function, immune responsiveness, stress, fatigue, control of viral infections and absorption of calcium and phosphorus, as well as those factors already mentioned.

Light

Although we have better indoor lighting than our ancestors, who had only candles and lamps to soften the darkness, we are still a long way from ideal conditions in our homes and workplaces. The trouble is we now spend more time indoors than ever before and we have almost cut ourselves off from the sun.

Electric lamps produce a light which is very distorted, with an excess of red rays. Even fluorescent lighting, which is better, comes nowhere near the true composition of natural ambient light. It has far too much yellow and green (cool colours).

Probably we allow ourselves insufficient internal illumination. In setting levels of 'adequate' lighting, only visual acuity has been

considered to date. In other words the amount of light supposedly
needed has been set by what is required to see, read and work
comfortably. No one, until recently, considered what is required,
physiologically speaking. It appears this is not the same at all.

The pineal gland

There is much speculation that the pineal gland is the source of
our sensitivity to light. This is a primitive organ found in the hind-

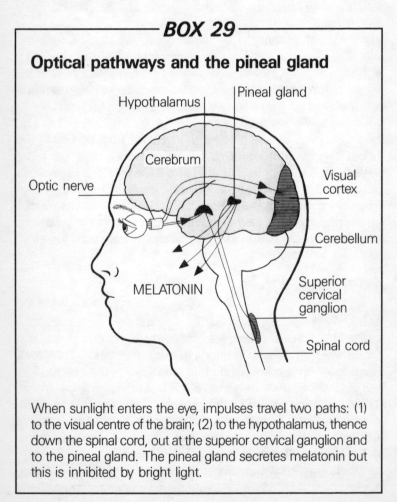

BOX 29

Optical pathways and the pineal gland

When sunlight enters the eye, impulses travel two paths: (1)
to the visual centre of the brain; (2) to the hypothalamus, thence
down the spinal cord, out at the superior cervical ganglion and
to the pineal gland. The pineal gland secretes melatonin but
this is inhibited by bright light.

brain, which is a survival of the 'third eye' of lizards and newts, though in humans it no longer connects with the exterior.

One theory is that it secretes a hormone called melatonin, thought to have a powerful effect on sleep, mood and reproductive cycles. It increases during the hours of darkness and subsides during the day. Presumably, SAD sufferers accumulate an excess of melatonin, or they are unduly sensitive to it.

Critics of this idea point to tests which showed that melatonin did not drop when humans were exposed to unexpected bright light in the middle of the night. But, say those who support the theory, this could be because we are so biologically adapted to our lifestyle, far removed from Nature, that a test like this is meaningless. In support, they will quote other experiments, where volunteers were made to sleep in darkened rooms during the day and work at night under bright sunlight equivalent until their natural adaptation was broken down. Then, when subjected to sudden bright light during the hours of (artificial) darkness, the melatonin levels did indeed drop significantly.

One thing that does seem certain is that light on the skin is not the important factor (as for vitamin D formation). It is light received via the eye that counts, though even blind people may show disturbances in day-night melatonin cycles. Probably the messages reach the pineal gland via the optical pathways in the brain (Box 29).

It is likely that other pathways are also involved. Single hormone control is nice in medical textbooks but matters are rarely that simple in life. We shall have to wait and see what turns up during the present intensive researches.

Treatment

Not surprisingly, the recommended treatment for SAD sufferers is light! Unfortunately, it is hard to subject this treatment to the rigours of double-blind challenge scrutiny, because it is not possible to disguise from the patient the fact that they are getting sunlight or its equivalent. Nevertheless, attempts to study the benefits objectively point to the fact that it is extremely helpful to those who suffer.

Obviously, real sunlight is best and one of the reasons that winter holidays abroad are becoming so popular in Britain is the fact that they are undoubtedly healthful and invigorating, allowing large doses of full-spectrum natural light, just when it is most scarce at home.

However, this is only a short-term solution. For more protracted treatments, some source of artificial sun equivalent is required. These are now available commercially at a reasonably economical price, though of course many times more costly than fluorescent so-called 'daylight' tubes. Details of a supplier in the UK is given in Useful Addresses at the end of the book.

Medical workers in this field suggest several hours a day of full-spectrum light. The most practical way to achieve this is to work near a high-intensity source but for many this is not practical. It may be necessary to divide the 'dose' between two sessions, night and morning. This way, up to six hours a day might be taken with advantage.

It goes without saying that patients should not self-diagnose and self-treat this condition. It is far better to find a doctor with the knowledge and skill required. At least two London hospitals are now working on the problem.

In the meantime, if you suspect SAD in your own case, draw back curtains and blinds, open windows as often as the weather allows and make a point of frequent walks in the open air. Even the pale wintery sun is thousands of times brighter than any artificial light source! Try to arrange two weeks' annual holiday, going south for the sun in the depths of winter, when experience tells you that you are at your lowest ebb. This should help recharge until spring comes along.

CHAPTER 12

Electricity

Planet Earth is a complex electrical environment. Even before Man set foot on it, never mind invented electricity generating machines, the whole globe was bathed in immense fields of charged particles, which in total power make our National Grid look like a glow-worm beside a nuclear explosion.

We are continually receiving bombardments of highly charged particles from the sun, the so-called Solar Wind. These sweep into our upper atmosphere where, fortunately for us, they are contained; though the upper layers become super-charged: the Ionosphere. Because of the Earth's polarity, these sheets of electrical energy only dip down to near ground level at the north and south poles and this effect gives rise to the aurorae. The Northern Lights (aurora borealis) are, in reality, nothing more than a giant electric storm. Observers who are close describe swishing and crackling noises, typical of electric discharges, and occasionally tingling and the smell of ozone, which is the familiar odour from electrical sparks.

If this isn't enough, then the whole rotating globe works rather like a giant dynamo, charging up the planet's very substance. Thus rocks have innate electricity, called piezo-electricity. It comes to the surface especially where there is volcanic and earthquake activity, and is the cause of a greenish glow often seen in the region of a recent earthquake.

Occasionally this 'rock electricity' escapes into the upper atmosphere, causing streamers or 'rays'; the well-known Andes glow is such a manifestation. Doubtless this accounts for a number of strange world-wide phenomena, phantom lights, apparitions etc. Even the flying saucer enthusiasts must concede that some sinister-looking lights in the sky have an entirely natural earth-bound origin.

St Elmo's Fire is an electrical effect which used to terrify our ancestors, especially sailors. A greenish glow surrounds objects, such as ships, buildings and even people under certain favourable atmospheric conditions. It is simply a harmless build-up of static electricity, but without the benefit of scientific knowledge it must have seemed a fearful, even diabolical, manifestation.

Then, of course, there is lightning in all its forms which, although intense, is a very minor effect in global terms and represents no more than a local build-up of static which then discharges itself.

Along came man

Then along came that inquisitive and inventive biped, homo sapiens (Man). By the time of the Ancient Greeks our species had discovered that rubbing amber with silk or fur produces static electricity (the Greek word for amber is elektron, hence electricity).

In the eighteenth century the Italian Volta (after whom the volt is named) discovered that alternate layers of copper and zinc discs, separated by brine-soaked cloths, gave rise to an electric current. The battery was born.

In the nineteenth century a Dutchman called Oersted discovered that a current in a wire has a magnetic field. In 1831 Michael Faraday realized the importance of the opposite effect: that if a coil of wire is rotated in a magnetic field, a current is produced. Thus the dynamo or generator was born.

This in turn led to other possibilities, such as the electric telegraph and Thomas Eddison's great boon, the electric light, which liberated Man from the shackles of night. It is impossible to overestimate the benefit of this simple advance, which lengthened the working day to a potential 24 hours and so speeded up Man's progress into the technological age. How much slower it would have been if we had all continued to down tools and books at sunset (there were lamps and candles, true, but these were not very good).

Finally, we arrive at the twentieth century, and today we have radios, TVs, dishwashers, vacuum cleaners, ovens, toasters, clocks and a whole host of gadgets powered by electricity, at work and in the home. Cables run everywhere, in walls, under floors and over our heads. We are literally surrounded by electricity, in a way which would have been unthinkable 150 years ago.

In an island like Britain, it is almost impossible to get away from electricity. Even if you went to the remoter parts of Scotland, you would have to avoid numerous hydro-electric plants in the mountains (not to mention Dounreay, the nuclear power station). Even then, you could not travel there by car (battery and ignition system) and the chances are you would have to leave behind your wrist-watch (battery quartz crystal model) and numerous other personal gadgets.

Our world has now altered. As a species, we evolved in natural electric fields. Possibly we are accustomed, biologically-speaking, to this background radiation. Yet we are now exposed to levels estimated conservatively at a million times greater. Some scientists put it as high as a hundred-million-fold increase in exposure. Isn't it strange, then, that nobody, until recently, asked the question: is it safe?

New and disturbing evidence suggests that indeed it is not.

What is life?

Well, all the written words since the dawn of time have not answered that question! But one thing is for sure: Life is electrical in nature. The difference between a dead cell and a live one is that the latter has an electric potential across its surface membrane. When the cell dies, that disappears.

We associate life, particularly in animals, with the ability to perceive and react to stimuli and — in higher forms, such as ourselves — the capacity to think. All this depends on electrical forces taking place in special tissues called the nervous system. It pervades our bodies but is consolidated especially in the organ we call the brain. Its functions are nothing more than a mass of electrical activity, but this can be measured outwardly by recording machines. Our very thoughts, feelings and identity thus have at least an electrical emanation, even if you believe implicitly in higher entities, such as the soul or spirit.

Logically, then, we can predict — without even first meeting a patient made sick by electricity — that to interfere with our body electricity, or distort its patterns with strong outside fields, will lead to trouble and feeling bad. It is important to remember here that the brain operates on very low electrical field potentials, far less than is found in a battery-powered wrist-watch, for example.

In fact, such patients are already coming to light. Too much electricity makes them ill. For them, the twentieth century is a nightmare, a living hell from which they cannot hope to escape, except by living on a remote island or in a safety oasis, screened from electromagnetic radiation by metal shields.

Far fetched? Read on . . .

Health hazard

Probably the most widely known electrical hazard is that associated with overhead electrical cables. Some studies have suggested it *might* be a cause of cancer, especially leukaemia in children.

One diligent UK practitioner documented many cases of suicide and found a much higher incidence than expected among people who live under or near overhead cables.

'Not enough proof,' say some scientists (especially those who work for the electricity board). 'Look at all the evidence,' say the opponents. The argument will rage on and will take years to settle; that's the way these things go.

But what we are talking about in this book are the much more immediate effects, which can easily be demonstrated here and now. Some patients are so intolerant of electricity that they can be wheeled (blindfold) towards a power cable and they will know when they come within the field because they begin to feel sick. Double-blind tests have been made, showing that some people can 'feel' an electric current switched on and off, because it provokes unpleasant reactions. Thus there is no way this can be a psychological invention.

If you doubt that, take the case of a Dorset village, with overhead cables right across it. The inhabitants began to feel sick (headache, blackouts etc.) when, unknown to them, the voltage was more than doubled. You'd have to put it down to mass hysteria, happening at the right time by unbelievable coincidence, to push aside this important evidence for the harmful effects of high-tension electricity (which is exactly what the Electricity Board boffins are doing!).

Make no mistake, the field around these overhead cables is fairly intense. If you take a fluorescent light tube under one on a dark night, it will begin to glow quite some distance from the cables. Is it surprising then, that biological effects are also felt at a distance?

Even more interesting; sensitivity to electrical fields can be made worse by metal in the mouth. This is especially true for allergy victims, who are often already debilitated. For some unlucky ones, the effect is nothing short of disastrous.

NASA (the American space agency) has a ruling that those working in strong electric fields must not have metal in their mouths. In other words, the effect is already known about, scientifically-speaking. Yet dentists tell us that something like four fifths of the adult population have metal in their mouths (usually mercury, but it may be nickel or aluminium). We live, daily, in electrical fields. Those under cables are especially exposed. So how can officialdom be so pompous and reassuring with its bland dismissals of the problem?

Allergics and electricity

My nurses know a lot about allergics and electricity. Frequently, when giving test injections, they get unpleasant static shocks. This happens far more often than in encounters with normal healthy individuals. Certain patients seem to be particularly bad in this respect and the effect can be most unpleasant, taxing the nurses' saintly devotion to the limit.

There is something special about allergic patients and electricity. Many of them seem able to cause damage to electrical equipment: kettles burn out, plugs explode, TV sets stop working, electric clocks go backwards. These and many other strange occurrences tell us that something out of the ordinary is happening. We don't as yet know what it is, but to scoff — just because you don't understand — is the hallmark of a fool. Sadly, there are plenty of these, even among so-called experts.

Some cases on record are truly remarkable. Certain individuals seem able to disrupt whole computer or telephone systems, merely by their presence. A number of strange individuals have been struck by lightning, many times over (see *The Guinness Book of Records*). There are even cases of people able to illuminate light bulbs by holding them in their hands.

Surprisingly, these curious individuals seem unharmed by their unusual electrical nature. The unfortunate fact, however, is that the majority of electrical sensitives are made ill by their experiences and, until recently, theirs was an unhappy lot. Nobody knew the cause of the trouble. They were, if you like, 'allergic to electricity'.

What to look for

As with true allergic phenomena, manifestations can be almost infinite, according to which part of the body is affected. However, those symptoms which give rise to the most concern are those connected with the nervous system. These include headaches, dizziness, weakness, poor concentration, insomnia and even nausea.

Typically, symptoms are worse near electrical equipment. Some patients know, for example, that when the television is switched on, they feel worse (I will avoid the obvious joke). Overhead cables are a hazard, but so are sub-stations and the small kerbside relay boxes. Some patients can 'feel' cables in the walls and floors at home.

Generally speaking, patients feel worse if they are in a field created by electrical appliances on either side. In a kitchen, the oven and fridge may be on one side and the kettle, radio and perhaps a microwave on the other, the poor housewife trapped between the two. A better arrangement is to have all appliances against one wall.

What to do

What does an electrically sensitive patient do to cope with our modern environment? As with all allergies, we say avoid it! That isn't easy, of course, though some are so ill they need to move to the country (avoiding overhead transmission lines), to get away from the worst urban concentrations.

If you can't avoid it, other steps may be necessary. One patient finds he is helped by wearing a copper plate on his back, wrapped in fabric to fit a wide belt. Others have tried metal screens, from foil to chicken wire, and some swear it helps. Science tells us, however, that to be truly effective, such a screen would need to be many inches thick, and clearly this is impracticable. My personal advice is to avoid this sort of approach until we understand the subject better. It is possible for metal to concentrate the field, instead of dissipating it. This would clearly be harmful.

Another approach is earthing. One way to do this, silly as it sounds, is to go outdoors barefoot. Contact with the earth will remove static build-up within the body. Feeling the grass between your toes may be more than a poetic way to feel good.

This is the exact opposite effect to our modern buildings, where synthetic carpets and dry air-conditioning help to build up considerable static charges. This contributes to the sick building syndrome (see page 62).

If outdoor earthing isn't practical, trail a wire round your wrist while sleeping and connect it to the central heating pipes or some other metal 'earth'. Standing barefoot on an earthed metal plate is another solution BUT BE CAREFUL. You must avoid the temptation to do this while handling electrical appliances. A comparatively minor accidental shock could well turn into a fatal one if you ignore this caution.

These tricks can easily become a habit, and patients swear by the beneficial results. It begins to sound cranky. I think it is better to keep these remedies for times when you really need them and not become psychologically dependant on such props.

Synthetic fabrics, of course, create static and are best avoided. Wear only cotton and silks where possible, especially next to the skin (underwear). Women might like to know that tights with a cotton gusset and soles to the feet are available. These will allow discharge to the floor, and reportedly feel better.

Keep a level head

Electrical sensitives are probably even more likely to develop a weird anti-social lifestyle than multi-allergics. It is vital to fight this tendency. However serious the problems, try to see the humorous side. Keep in contact with your environment, don't run and hide from it. In any case, you should remember that electrical fields within your home are, if anything, worse than those in a motor car or walking down the street, so moping indoors isn't logical.

New researches have suggested it may be possible to 'neutralize' electrical fields with certain frequencies, specific to the patient, rather like the neutralizing 'drops' of Miller's method. The patient doesn't need to swallow the remedy; simply to hold or carry a resonator of the right frequency may be sufficient.

Beyond these tips, the only approach to electrical problems is unburdening — that is, the correction of diet, lack of stress, rest and vitamins to strengthen the biological resistance of your body.

CHAPTER 13

Geopathic stress

Finally, we come to one of the most bizarre but exciting new concepts in the art of healing. If you think the last chapter was rather startling and strange, you will find this topic entirely off the medical map. This is unchartered territory, scientifically-speaking, and only a handful of dauntless souls have investigated it, very few of them doctors. Nevertheless, I bring it to your attention because personally I believe it is a valid and important field; I have cases to support it and I think it will grow in recognition.

I am talking about Geopathic Stress, the idea that there are certain places on the earth's surface that are definitely harmful to life. The theory is that if you happen to live on such a location or, even worse, sleep on one, then your health may suffer until you correct it.

Ancient wisdom

From time immemorial there has been the belief that there are good and bad places to be. Often good places were considered blessed, such as sites of ancient temples, and megalithic circles. The bad spots, not unnaturally, were said to be evil and associated with bad spirits. Some were associated with stories of misdeeds or catastrophe as the origin of the bad feelings, rather like a haunting.

Sometimes the ancients took this further, and it has been discovered that many of their sites (dwellings, temples or stone circles) actually lie in long straight lines, stretching in some cases for over a hundred miles across country. These lines often bear no relation to geographical or astronomical features and the only way to explain them so far has been the suggestion that these artefacts are following invisible lines of energy: so-called ley lines.

Animals too

It isn't just humans. Country folk can tell you that there are certain places which animals avoid instinctively. Many farmers have, or know of, some field or corner of a field, where cattle cannot graze safely. The beasts simply become inexplicably sick and have to be moved.

As rural areas have receded and been covered with housing, many of these sites are now lived on by human beings.

One such place called to my attention has an unusually high incidence of cancer, multiple sclerosis and early death due to heart disease. It so happens that this is a modern housing estate on what was farming land within living memory. By chance, an old man was found who remembered the area. He at once referred to it as 'the bad lands' because livestock could not be grazed there. Cattle became sick and died, without any obvious cause.

Do you think this is just a coincidence or a flight of fancy? The more pertinent question, for those living in such a place, is: can you afford to take the risk with your own health and that of your family?

Geomagnetic energy

The earth's geomagnetic flux is an energy field to which we are all subject. It is certainly tied up with the piezo-electricity effect discussed in the previous chapter. Animals seem to depend a great deal on this magnetism. For example, homing pigeons with a tiny magnet strapped to their heads (to cancel out the earth's field), become hopelessly lost and cannot find their way home.

It was once assumed (with incredible scientific stupidity) that Man was somehow unaffected by this field. However, early space flights showed that, once separated from it, astronauts became sick and disorientated. Now rocket vehicles carry a built-in magnetic field, to match that of the earth, and the problem has been cured.

It seems quite logical, therefore, to assume that any diminution or intensification of the field will produce harmful levels of radiation, which in turn will lead to illness. Is there any way this can happen? Apparently there is.

Along the lines of geological faults, the 'rays' may be funnelled towards the surface. This intensifies the field. Conversely, underground streams, caverns and mineral deposits can reduce it. Underground water is particularly important in this respect, yet surface water seems to have no effect. The problem is worst where two underground streams cross, which takes place, of course, at different levels. Similarly, any pair of hazards coinciding will greatly increase the risk.

Just how important this phenomenon is can be gauged from the section on cancer below, but first, a word about dowsing.

The art of dowsing

A lot of evidence for the findings reported in this chapter comes from dowsing. Unfortunately, this venerable art does not enjoy a favourable reputation in the UK, though on the Continent it is highly regarded and widely used by both doctors and scientists. In Germany, for example, not noted for trivial, time-wasting pursuits, even government officials will turn to it, when necessary (and get results). Over 3,000 doctors are known to call in a dowser when there are real difficulties with a case.

Roche, the well-known international pharmaceutical firm, uses dowsers to locate the large supplies of water needed for their chemical processes. Their excuse? It works!

Huge North American oil companies often employ what they coyly term BPM (bio-physical method — in other words, dowsing). Make no mistake, they are not in the game of wasting money on mumbo-jumbo with no results.

Most people have heard of water-divining, which is dowsing for underground water, but it is possible to dowse also for the whereabouts of lost objects, people, minerals — in fact, anything you set your mind on. There are far too many documented cases of dowsers turning up finds in remote and unlikely places for these to be mere coincidence. The method may not be infallible but it certainly WORKS.

My first contact with dowsing for geopathic stress was at a medical meeting in Dublin. A case was cited of a severely ill child who failed to respond to conventional therapy. In desperation the parents had called in a dowser, who discovered the house contained several 'black spots', and one of these was exactly over the child's bed. As soon as the bed was relocated the child began to recover. Could this be the reason, I began to ask myself, why some of our cases fail, despite the very best treatment?

Since then I have heard there are hundreds of thousands of such stories. Now a growing number of properly qualified UK doctors are turning to dowsing when cases won't respond. This means being subjected to the scoffing and scorn of colleagues but, for doctors who really care and genuinely want to try to help their patients, this is no deterrent.

Findings that are hard to ignore

Beginning in 1929, Gustav Freiherr von Pohl, a talented German dowser, began to study the causal link between earth radiation and cancer. He devised a scale of force from 1-16 and considered anything above 9 to be cancer-inducing. He dowsed the village of Vilsbiburg, marking on a map all the zones which had a rating of 9 or higher. Then came the incredible discovery: after comparing hospital records with his map he found that all 54 cases who had died of cancer, since records began, had their beds on one of his zones. Of course there was scepticism so he did the whole experiment over again in another village, Grafenau, with exactly the same result. This time there were 16 such deaths, *all sleeping over danger zones.*

His findings were subsequently published by the Central Committee for Cancer Research and presented at a medical congress in Munich in 1930, where they attracted much interest. Who knows — if it hadn't been for the rise of Adolph Hitler, who suppressed von Pohl's work at this time because the redoubtable baron was an outspoken critic of Nazism, it might already be part of the standard medical canon.

Dr Hager, in Stettin, President of the Scientific Association of Medical Doctors (no crank by any means), went about investigating matters the other way round. He studied 5,348 cancer deaths recorded since 1910, dowsing their homes. Incredibly, he found that every single one had been exposed to strong earth radiation over a number of years. Some houses were so dangerous that many cancer deaths had taken place in them.

In the late 1970s an Austrian maths teacher Käthe Bachler concluded that children with learning difficulties may be exposed to harmful rays. In what was the most important study ever undertaken into earth radiation as a causative factor in disease, she studied over 11,000 cases and 3,000 homes in over 14 countries. Once again it showed that cancer only occurs over strong earth radiation. But, more importantly from our point of view, it showed conclusively that 95 per cent of children with problems slept or had their school desk over strong radiation (underground streams crossing etc.).

Typical symptoms included tiredness, lack of appetite, moodiness, lack of concentration, learning difficulties, disruptive or hyperactive behaviour and poor sleep. Does this sound like maladaptation? Of course; that's why this chapter is here.

Dr Manfred Curry, in Germany, dowsed the houses of several cancer patients. Without knowing anything whatever about the patients, he was able to say, from the position of the rays, where the cancer was located and in every case he was correct. In one bed, where the said rays crossed over the pelvic area of the sleeping person, two women had died of cancer of the uterus! He took several sceptical doctors along as witnesses. Needless to say, they were pretty startled by the demonstration.

There is more evidence. But anyone who doesn't think earth radiation needs to be taken seriously, after reading the above, is probably the kind to jump out of an aircraft at 10,000 feet without a parachute, claiming it is safe. It is doubtful if more words would be persuasive.

Other geopathic stresses

Dr Manfred Curry dowsed the existence of a series of lines crossing the earth in an interconnecting grid, now known as the Curry Net. The lines are about 3.5 metres apart and alternately charging and discharging (positive and negative). Where two lines of the same polarity cross is thought to be particularly harmful.

Dr Ernst Hartmann is father of yet another energy net, known as the Hartmann Grid or Global Grid. It seems to be of cosmic origin and varies with sun spots, earth magnetism, atmospheric conditions and phases of the moon. The lines are 2-3 metres apart, run north-south and, once again, the intersections are the sites of maximum intensity.

The Curry net lies diagonally to the Hartmann Grid.

Allergy and geopathic stress

What has geopathic stress to do with allergies? Two things. First of all, the symptoms of geopathic stress can easily be mistaken for maladaptation. Those most commonly quoted include insomnia and sleep disturbance, cramps, cold feet, tingling in the arms and legs, grinding of teeth, sweating, shivering, fatigue and lethargy, feeling run down and 'exhausted', depression, nervous tension, mood changes, aggression, lack of appetite, pallor and resistance to medical treatment.

These are symptoms of a body under stress. This may be important. If you are trying to find a food allergy and the real cause is geopathic stress then, naturally, you will fail.

Secondly, if an allergy case is not responding, despite every endeavour and the successful identification and elimination of allergies, geopathic stress may be the reason.

Thus an arthritis or eczema case, for example, who does not improve despite careful diet, may benefit from moving the bed or somehow neutralizing the earth radiation, as described in the next section.

It is not that attention to geopathic stress will preclude the need for other sorts of medical treatment, but simply that it may allow it to work when previously it did not.

What can be done?

As with all environmental hazards, the best method is to avoid the stress. However, you may not know that you are subject to such a hazard. If you suspect it for any reason, you can always try moving your bed to see if you feel any better.

Check the history of the house you are living in, if it isn't brand new. Sometimes there have been many illnesses among past occupants that may give you a clue.

Clearly it would be sensible to hire the services of a dowser. As in any profession, some are good and some are not. Try to make contact with someone competent through The British Society of Dowsers. The address is given in the appendix.

If it is established there is radiation in your home, especially at the site of the bed, you had better do something. It may be possible to relocate the bed or change sleeping rooms. If it is not practical to do this for some reason, you may like to try neutralizing the rays. But it would be prudent to have the dowser pronounce the bed clear before you assume this has worked.

I do not intend to give a comprehensive guide here on what to do about earth rays, but I will give you some suggestions which you can follow up.

- Crystals or coils located in specific spots in your house (these spots have to be dowsed out).

- Metal plates, earthed, under your mattress.

- Driving iron rods into the ground at the point where the rays enter and leave.

- Placing specific precious stones where the rays enter and leave.

- A 6-9 inch high copper pyramid, placed under the bed at the level of the solar plexus (in Germany hundreds of thousands of these pyramids are sold). The pyramid needs discharging regularly, by running under the tap.

- A 1 metre length of copper wire, laid in a ring under the mattress, with a 10cm gap open to the north.

According to T. E. Peltonen, a Finnish author, such devices give about an 80 per cent success rate. This is good odds for allergies, but you may feel, if you are frightened of cancer, that this isn't good enough. *The safest rule is always to avoid the radiation altogether.*

Further reading

In a book of this size it is impossible to give more than an outline of the facts in relation to allergy and environmental medicine. It is vital that the sufferer learns as much as possible about the subject and reading widely the works of many different authors is the way to do this.

Apart from one cookbook, books written by other than competent qualified physicians are not included. Only those who practise medicine and understand the wider health implications of allergy are recommended. Much misleading and frankly hazardous information abounds in books by enthusiastic amateurs who think that recovering from their own illness makes them an expert. This still leaves plenty of reading matter!

Included is a section of books which you might care to recommend to your doctor, if you can get him or her interested in the issue.

General nutrition

Davies, S. and Stewart, A., *Nutritional Medicine: The Drug-free Guide to Better Family Health*, Pan Books, London (1987)

Lesser, M., *Nutrition and Vitamin Therapy*, Thorsons, Wellingborough (1985)

Newbold, H. L., *Meganutrients for your Nerves*, Berkeley Publishing Corporation, New York (1975)

Pfeiffer, C. C., *Zinc and Other Micronutrients*, Keats, Connecticut (1978)

Wright, J. V., *Dr Wright's Book of Nutritional Therapy*, Rodale Press, Pennsylvania (1979)

Chemical allergy

Mackarness, R., *Chemical Victims*, Pan Books, London (1980)
Randolph, T. G., *Human Ecology and Susceptibility to the Chemical Environment*, Charles C. Thomas, Springfield, Illinois (1962)
Randolph, T. G. and Moss, R. W., *Allergies — Your Hidden Enemy*, Turnstone Press, Wellingborough (1981)

Food allergy

Food Watch, *The Food Watch Alternative Cookbook* (1984) (see Useful addresses).
Mackarness, R., *Not All in the Mind*, Pan Books, London (1985)
Miller, J. B., *Relief At Last*, Charles C. Thomas, Springfield, Illinois (1987)
Mumby, K., *The Food Allergy Plan*, Allen & Unwin, London (1985)
Workam, E., Alun Jones, V. and Hunter, J. O., *The Allergy Diet*, Martin Dunitz, London (1985)

Children

Crook. W. G., *Tracking Down Hidden Food Allergies*, Professional Books, P.O. Box 3494, Jackson, Tennessee 38301, USA
Feingold, B. F., *Why Your Child is Hyperactive*, Random House, New York (1974)
Rapp, D. J., *Allergies and the Hyperactive Child*, Thorsons (1988)
Rapp, D. J., *Allergies and Your Family*, Sterling Publishing, New York (1980)

Candida

Crook, W. G., *The Yeast Connection*, Professional Books, P.O. Box 3494, Jackson, Tennessee 38301, USA (1984)
Truss, O., *The Missing Diagnosis*, P.O. Box 26508, Birmingham, Alabama 35226, USA (1983)

For the doctor

Breneman, J. C., *Basics of Food Allergy*, Charles C. Thomas, Springfield, Illinois (1978)

Brostoff, J. and Challacombe, S. J., *Food Allergy and Intolerance*, Baillière Tindall, Eastbourne (1987)

Dickey, L. D. (Ed.), *Clinical Ecology*, Charles C. Thomas, Springfield, Illinois (1976)

Miller, J. B., *Food Allergy: Provocative Testing and Injection Therapy*, Charles C. Thomas, Springfield, Illinois (1972)

Philpott, W. H. and Kalita, D. K., *Brain Allergies: The Psychonutrient Connection*, Keats (1980)

Geopathic stress

Gordon, Rolf, *Are You Sleeping in a Safe Place?*, Dulwich Health Society (see Useful addresses)

Von Pohl, Gustav Freiherr, *Earth Currents*, Ilse Pope, 1 Garry Close, Romford, Essex RM1 4EA.

General

Mandell, M. and Scanlon, L. W., *Dr Mandell's Five-Day Allergy Relief System*, Crowell, New York (1979)

Mumby, K., *Allergies — What Everyone Should Know*, Allen & Unwin, London (1986)

Of course, the list is far from complete but the many references contained in each of these works should lead you on to much more of interest. Some of the books are now out of print, but you may be able to find them at the public library. Bon appetit!

Useful addresses

To conclude, here is a list of some addresses that you may find useful. These are accurate at the time of going to press. Probably the most useful of all, as a source of information for doctors and public alike, is the first. But please remember it is a charity and make some donation if you want help or advice.

Action Against Allergy
43, The Downs
London SW20 8HG

Offers considerable support and advice to allergy sufferers. Details of organic food suppliers and low-risk household products. Scientific papers available to medical practitioners. Large book department for sale or loan.

The British Society of Dowsers
Sycamore Cottage
Tamley
Hastingleigh
Ashford
Kent TN25 5HW

They have members all over the country who undertake to dowse for harmful earth rays. Dowsers may charge anything from a cup of tea to £30.00 for a survey.

The Dulwich Health Society
130 Gipsy Hill
London SE19 1PL

A non-profit-making society whose aims are to co-ordinate and
disseminate research from all over the world into geopathic stress.

Food Watch
Butts Pond Industrial Estate
Sturminster Newton
Dorset DT10 1AZ

An example of a small business supplying organic and special foods
for allergics.

Foresight Association
Mrs Peter Barnes
The Old Vicarage
Church Lane
Witley
Godalming
Surrey GU8 5PN

Advice on diet, nutrition and allergies for parents-to-be — *before
conception*.

Henry Doubleday Research Association
National Centre for Organic Gardening
Ryton-on-Dunsmore
Coventry CV8 3LG

Research into organic farming methods. Publishes a book of organic
growers and suppliers (which unfortunately goes out of date very
rapidly).

Hyperactive Children's Support Group
71 Whyke Lane
Chichester
West Sussex PO19 2LD

Advice to parents of hyperactive children, including diets, vitamins,
etc. Publishes a newsletter. Many sub-groups: there should be one
active near you.

Myalgic Encephalomyelitis Association
P.O. Box 8
Stanford-Le-Hope
Essex SS17 8EX

Advice for ME sufferers, though guarded about the validity of the nutritional, environmental and allergy approach as outlined in this book.

National Society for Research into Allergy
P.O. Box 45
Hinckley
Leicestershire L10 1JY

Also considerable help to allergy sufferers, though rather conventional and limited in outlook, advice and treatments.

Sanity
63 Coal Park Road
Twickenham
Middlesex TW1 1HT

Promotes knowledge concerning the nutritional and environmental factors in mental illness.

Schizophrenia Association of Great Britain
Tyr Twr
Llanfair Hall
Caernarvon
North Wales

Supports research into the physical causes of this distressing mental illness.

Society for Environmental Therapy
3 Atherton Road
Ipswich
Suffolk IP4 2LD

A scientific society for doctors, scientists and lay people who are concerned about the effects of environmental factors on health.

Soil Association
86 Colston St
Bristol BS1 5BB

Watchdogs of environmental poisons, engaged in studying pesticide effects and disseminating knowledge concerning chemical agricultural methods and its hazards. Publishes booklets. Vets organic produce, ensuring it deserves the label as such.

Specialist Lighting Distributors
S.M.L.
Unit 4, Wye Trading Estate
London Road
High Wycombe
Buckinghamshire HP11 1LH

York Medical and Nutritional Laboratory
126 Acomb Road
York YO2 4EY

Provides a cytotoxic allergy test service, as well as general advice on allergy and nutrition.

Index

(page numbers in italics refer to tables)

allowance (RDA), 67
rhinitis, 23, 53
rice
    in diabetic diets, 42
    flour, 44
Rinkel, H., 17
rodent urine, 58
rotation diet, 45-50
Royal Free Disease (see) post-
    viral fatigue syndrome
rye flour, 44

sago, 44
St Anthony's fire, 56
St Elmo's fire, 119-20
St Vitus' dance, 56
seasonal affective disorder
    (SAD), 114-18
    treatment, 117-18
selenium, 68, 71, 72
    in mercury allergy, 112
sensitization, 18
serial end-point skin titration,
    78-80
sheep's milk, 43
shellfish allergy, 29
Sick Building Syndrome, 62
smoking, 33, 35
solar radiation, 115
Soothil, I., 14
soya flour, 44
'Stone-Age diet', 31, 32
strawberry allergy, 29
stress, 17, 52, 53
sub-lingual provocation and
    neutralization method, 80
sugar
    allergy, 29
    in Candida albicans
        infection, 94
    omitting from diet, 43
sulphur dioxide, 51
symptoms of allergy, 22, 24-7,
    (see also) withdrawal
    symptoms
    food sensitivity, 30

T-cells, 103

Tapnui 'Flu (see) post-viral
    fatigue syndrome
target organs, 22-4
The Pulse Test, 26
threshold dose, 16, 18, 19
thrush, 87
tobacco, 33
total body load, 52-3
total environmental control
    unit, 83
trace elements, 68
tranquillizers, 74
Truss, O., 87

urea-formaldehyde, 58

vaccination, 13
vaginal thrush, 96
Vega machine, 81-2, 109
vegetarian diet, 39
vitamins, 66-8
    dosage, 71-2
    imbalance, 66
    and immune system, 69-72
    in mercury allergy, 112
    therapy, 72-4
    in treatment of post-viral
        fatigue syndrome, 104
von Pohl, G.F., 129

wheat,
    allergy, 8, 29, 40
    in cooking, 44
    omitting from diet, 43
    substitutes, 44
white blood cells, 13, 52
withdrawal symptoms, 20, 26,
    41
woolly brain syndrome, 24

yeast, 93-5
    allergy, 29
    omitting from diet, 43
yogurt, 95

zinc, 68, 70, 72, 73, 74
    in mercury allergy, 112